Knee Arthrography

Knee Arthrography

Dennis J. Stoker

F.R.C.P., F.R.C.R.

Consultant Radiologist
Royal National Orthopaedic
and St. George's Hospitals
London
Director of Radiological Studies
The Institute of Orthopaedics
London

1980
SPRINGER-SCIENCE+BUSINESS MEDIA, B.V.

© 1980 D.J.Stoker
Originally published by Chapman and Hall in 1980
Softcover reprint of the hardcover 1st edition 1980

ISBN 978-0-412-21860-6

British Library Cataloguing in Publication Data

Stoker, Dennis J
  Knee arthrography.

  1. Knee–Radiography
  I. Title
  617'.582'07572   RC932   80–40619

  ISBN 978-0-412-21860-6   ISBN 978-1-4899-3160-3 (eBook)
  DOI 10.1007/978-1-4899-3160-3

Contents

TO ANNE

Foreword

Of the joints of the body commonly afflicted by serious pathology the knee is the most accessible. Because it is so accessible drastic treatment may be undertaken prematurely and incorrectly. This does not threaten life but may cause permanent morbidity.

Dr Stoker has set about examining this joint in depth as a radiologist. As a direct result the surgeon will be helped to make a correct diagnosis and avoid pitfalls, by a diagnostic procedure that is of little inconvenience to a patient. Arthrography is not new but a fresh appraisal is timely.

This is not to suggest that there can be any slackening in clinical examination, or that other methods of examination do not have a place. But there are knee joint problems, particularly in teenage girls, in which a clinical diagnosis is very difficult, but must be made exactly.

Arthrography must be accepted as a very useful method of examination of the knee joint and an essential one in certain circumstances. More radiologists should be interested in undertaking this examination and surgeons should ask for it.

E.L. Trickey, F.R.C.S.
Royal National Orthopaedic Hospital
Stanmore

Preface

A growing interest in arthrography of the knee has been evident in the United Kingdom during the last 5 to 7 years; the advantages offered by the technique have been appreciated by radiologists, orthopaedic surgeons and especially all those involved in the practice of sports medicine. Although the use of arthrography is more widespread in North America and parts of continental Europe, this is not necessarily a reflection of a lesser awareness of its benefits, but rather of a general shortage of qualified radiologists and a need, therefore, to apply a series of priorities to the radiological service commitment in the United Kingdom. I am, in fact, often approached by radiologists who wish to set up an arthrographic service and need advice about technique, in addition to those who have started to undertake knee arthrograms and have met difficulties in the achievement of a high standard in radiographic quality.

Many articles have been published on various facets of the arthrographic procedure, but few manuals on the whole technique of arthrography. This is not to neglect the outstanding monograph by Ricklin, Rüttiman and del Buono, to whom I, and many other established arthrographers, owe a tremendous debt. In an attempt to answer some of the questions posed, I have produced this monograph. A detailed technique is described, from which the emergent arthrographer may deviate, as his experience grows, by adaptation to meet his own local facilities and his increasing proficiency. The illustrations of arthrograms cannot and, indeed, should not be comprehensive; sufficient illustrations have been included to cover most of the routine and common difficult areas.

This book is intended primarily for radiologists. It can be read with benefit by the other member of the arthrographic team, the radiographer, for whom arthrography supplies an involvement greater than most other contrast examinations. The satisfaction of the examination, as with many other radiological techniques, lies in the solution of a clinical problem to the benefit of the patient. The radiologist who achieves any success with arthrography should, therefore, find that a closer relationship as a member of the diagnostic team leads to better sequent information from the referring clinician. The orthopaedic surgeon who reads this book, and I hope that many will, can thereby appreciate what follows his signing of the request from, and the care taken by the radiologist to ensure that the information in his report is based upon accurate observation in an impeccable technique.

Acknowledgements

It would not be possible to mention the names of all those, without whose help and encouragement, the production of this book would not have been possible. To those whose names I omit, I apologize in advance.

I am grateful to my radiological colleagues at the Royal National Orthopaedic Hospital, Dr Ronald Murray and Dr Malcolm Chapman, for encouraging me to take up this investigation and for making it possible for me to attend other centres where the technique was already well established. I owe a great debt to Robert Freiberger, M.D., of the Hospital for Special Surgery, New York, for his help and advice and for convincing me of the great value of the investigation on the basis of his extensive experience. I must thank also Paul Butt, M.D., previously of Montreal General Hospital, for easily convincing me that the fluoroscopic spot-film technique was superior to the purely radiographic methods in earlier use.

I am grateful to all orthopaedic surgeons and other clinicians who have referred their patients to me for arthrography; in particular, I must thank Mr Lorden Trickey, F.R.C.S., who was my primary support in the early days when the technique was evolving, quality was variable and accuracy was very much less predictable than at present. The ability to correlate the radiographic findings with clinical, arthroscopic and operative findings, and to discuss the studies subsequently, is an indication of team-work from which the patient can only benefit.

The success of the technique described here depends primarily on the radiographers, who may remember nostalgically the relatively quiet times in the department before knee arthrography took off. I must thank especially Mr Bill Stripp, M.S.R., Superintendent Radiographer at the Town Hospital of the Royal National Orthopaedic Hospital, for his unfailing good humour in establishing and maintaining the radiographic quality, and for his inventiveness in the solution of technical problems. At the Country branch of the Hospital, my thanks are due to Miss Mary Manhire, M.S.R., Superintendent Radiographer until 1977, whose help was invaluable in the early years. My thanks are also due to Mrs Ann Smith, M.S.R., now Superintendent Radiographer at the Country branch of the Hospital, but earlier, the radiographer mainly assigned to help in the establishment of an examination of diagnostic quality with equipment that was far from suited to the task. To all other radiographers, past and present, at both branches of the Hospital, I am grateful for tolerance and good humour, in addition to the technical skill one has come to take for granted.

Although we employed no permanent full-time junior medical staff in radiology, many part-time and temporary registrars have been involved in this work. I am grateful to them, both for relieving me of the burden of physically having to undertake every knee arthrogram myself and for teaching me the various problems experienced by those in training in learning this technique. Of the sometime senior registrars, I am particularly grateful to Drs Peter Renton, Henry Loose, Andrew Fulton and Nan Mitchell.

Aseptic techniques cannot be performed without nursing assistance, so my gratitude goes to Sister Eve Hunter and Sisters, Staff Nurses and Nurses at both branches of the Hospital, too numerous to mention.

The photographic illustrations have been undertaken with great care and expertise by the Medical Photography Department of the Institute of Orthopaedics and my special thanks go to Mrs Uta Boundy and Miss Hellena Swire for the reproduction of many radiographs of small size.

I should also like to thank Miss Francesca Marcus of the Royal National Orthopaedic Hospital, Stanmore and Miss Rosalind Nobbs of the Middlesex Hospital School of Radiography, for their help with a number of illustrations.

A number of drawings have been made by Mr Alan Jones of the Educational Technology Unit, St George's Hospital Medical School; I am extremely grateful to him for sparing the time to execute these explanatory anatomical drawings.

To my secretary, Veronika Aurens, my thanks are due for the typing of the manuscript and for generally keeping everything, including myself, in order.

1 Arthrography of the knee

1.1 Introduction

The knee is one of the most frequently injured joints in the body, being the most mobile and least stable of the weight-bearing joints. Most athletic injuries to the knee involve the soft tissue elements; ligaments, menisci, synovium and articular cartilage. It is, therefore, not surprising that plain film radiography is of limited value in the diagnosis of such injuries. In most cases, an experienced clinician will be able to diagnose a meniscal lesion from the history and his physical examination. However, clinical examination is demonstrably fallible, because some meniscal lesions do not produce characteristic symptoms or signs. This occurs for a variety of reasons, e.g. a clinical sign dependent on the displacement of a meniscal fragment may be negative either because the tear is too small to allow displacement in the clinical test or too large, so that the fragment is permanently displaced.

The need for greater diagnostic accuracy is supported by observations (Tapper and Hoover, 1969; Johnson *et al.*, 1974) that adverse sequelae follow the removal of a normal meniscus and that therefore a meniscus should be excised only when it is abnormal and the cause of symptoms.

Knee arthrography is a valuable adjunct to clinical examination in the diagnosis of internal derangement of the knee, particularly in the identification of damage to the menisci.

1.2 Historical

Arthrography of the knee is not a new investigation, despite the interest shown in it in recent years. The first arthrographic examination was reported by Werndorff and Robinson at the fourth German Orthopaedic Conference in 1905, just 10 years after the discovery of X-rays; on this occasion air was employed as the contrast medium. A year later, arthrography employing oxygen was reported (Hoffa, 1906; Rauenbusch, 1906). In a paper in 1926, Bernstein and Arens favoured the use of carbon dioxide, because it was non-irritant and readily absorbed. Little further progress was made until the 1930s, when positive-contrast arthrography was introduced. Further spread of the technique was probably hampered by the relative toxicity of the early iodinated media. By 1948, however, Lindblom was able to report his results in over 4000 positive-contrast examinations, demonstrating that the technique was diagnostically accurate.

During the period 1930 to 1936, Bircher and Oberholzer published a number of papers covering over 1200 cases. In their paper of 1934, based on 700 arthrographic examinations, they stressed the overall value of the double-contrast technique they had introduced. A number of papers were published after 1940 from English, American, German and Scandinavian centres, but still indicated a variety of contrast techniques.

Cullen and Chance (1943) introduced the next advance with the horizontal beam technique, which was subsequently modified by the use of a fulcrum by Meschan and McGaw (1947). The popularity of double-contrast arthrography increased thereafter (van der Berg and Crèvecoeur, 1951) and was refined and improved by combination with stress films, using a horizontal beam and an increased focus–film distance by Andrén and Wehlin (1960). This technique, further refined by Freiberger (Freiberger *et al.*, 1966), produced excellent diagnostic results. With the improvement of fluoroscopic equipment, clear visualization of the meniscus on the television screen followed, and this technique, coupled with spot films, was described in the excellent monograph of Ricklin *et al.* (1971) and in North America by Butt and McIntyre (1969). This remains the radiographic technique presently employed in most centres, although modifications of detail have evolved. Nevertheless, Tegtmeyer *et al.* (1979) have reported that a similar degree of diagnostic accuracy can be expected whether the single- or double-contrast method is employed.

In the United Kingdom, in contradistinction to Europe and North America, arthrography of the knee has been accepted less readily by both clinicians and radiologists, although its use is increasing. The reasons for the slow adoption of this useful diagnostic technique are probably two-fold.

(1) In this country, the long tradition of the over-riding supremacy of clinical signs and the virtual absence of objective studies relating pre-operative diagnosis to the findings at meniscectomy have suggested, until relatively recently, that no need for ancillary diagnostic methods existed.

(2) The relatively low standing of radiology, compared to North America and Scandinavia, is coupled with, or indeed has resulted in, a shortage of trained radiologists in this country. As a consequence, new time-consuming techniques do not tend to be introduced without evidence of increasing demands from the surgeons or other clinicians.

The majority of meniscal injuries are accurately diagnosed by clinical examination. It is not yet the case in Britain, as it seems to be in certain centres in the United States, that knee arthrotomy is not performed without prior arthrography and/or arthroscopy. Nevertheless, arthrography provides a valuable and accurate investigation, where physical signs are minimal or contradictory. The appreciation of the short-comings of clinical signs in the diagnosis of meniscal lesions has emphasized the need for arthrography to be practised more widely in the United Kingdom.

1.3 Positive-contrast media: historical

In the 1930s, positive-contrast media of the diiodized ('iodoxyl') type were employed.

Burman *et al.* (1932) injected 10 ml lipiodol into the human knee, noting severe pain from about 3 h after the injection diminishing gradually but not disappearing for 2 to 11 days. Clinical evidence of a chemical synovitis was present. They concluded that lipiodol should never be used intra-articularly.

Lindblom (1948) used 10 ml 35 per cent perabrodil, which caused a late irritation in 5 per cent of cases, or 4 ml uroselectan B plus novocaine, which caused pain for a few seconds following injection, but no late symptoms. He commented on the improved accuracy of positive-contrast arthrography, in comparison to gas arthrograms, in his own department.

1.4 Positive-contrast media currently available

In a double-contrast examination it is necessary to use both a positive- and a negative-contrast medium. The positive-contrast media available are all salts of iodinated organic acids, which have usually been elaborated for intravascular use. The objective in arthrography is not that the medium should mix with a body fluid, but coat the synovial lining of the joint. The qualities required, and the technique, have much more in common with double-contrast techniques used in the gastro-intestinal tract, although it is not desirable to inject non-soluble matter, such as barium, into a joint.

The function of a good medium is to produce a thin, but dense, opacification of the lining surface of the joint. The degree of opacification depends upon the iodine content of the medium and the depth of its surface layer which is mainly dependent upon its viscosity. Other local conditions, known, such as the presence of synovitis or effusion, or unknown, affect the final result. Available contrast media include sodium and meglumine salts or a mixture of both. Sodium salts cause greater chemical synovitis and discomfort and may cause pain when injected outside the joint. Occasional radiologists use sodium diatrizoate 45 per cent, and if the patient experiences pain, know that the needle is no longer in the synovial cavity; this is not a technique that can possibly be recommended.

A list (not necessarily comprehensive) of suitable media is shown in Table 1.1.

The contrast medium is absorbed directly from the synovial surface. Undoubted-

Table 1.1

Proprietary name	Manufacturer	Approved name	Wt/vol	Iodine content (mg/ml)	Viscosity at 37°C (mPa s)	Osmolality (mOsm/litre)
Conray 280	May & Baker	meglumine iothalamate	60%	280	4	1570
Urografin 310M (65%) (Angiografin)	Schering Chemicals	meglumine diatrizoate	65%	305	5.1	1060
Dimer X	May & Baker	meglumine iocarmate	60%	280		1040
Amipaque	Nyegaard	metrizamide		280	5.0 (depending upon desired concentration)	456*

*mOsm/kg water.

ly, in every case, some leaks out through the needle puncture into the periarticular tissues and, in a proportion of patients, the synovium may not be intact as a consequence of capsular rupture. Such absorbed medium is excreted by the kidneys. The absorption of the contrast medium not only means that positive contrast is lost in a finite time, but blurring and haziness of the articular margins occurs, producing a less acceptable picture. Fortunately, a competent arthrographer is able to complete the examination within 10 to 15 min of injection, in which time no significant reduction in film quality has occurred.

Consideration of a medium with slower absorption may be worth while for various reasons, e.g. in a training programme where greater time is needed by the student, where the initial films are spoilt for some reason, and in the presence of synovitis. As it is clearly not possible on many occasions to predict delays or problems that may arise, one would have to use a long-acting contrast technique as a routine. We have not found this necessary. Several contrast techniques of this type have been described.

Meglumine Iocarmate ('Dimer X') has been described by Roebuck (1977) as superior to equivalent monomeric compounds, because of its delayed absorption. We have used Dimer X with our standard technique but, like Grech (1977) in hip arthrography, we have not found any slight advantage to outweigh the greatly increased cost. Indeed, we have not had problems with monomeric compounds that would necessitate a change. Similarly, we have not found the need for routine addition of adrenaline to the contrast medium, as advocated by Hall (1974).In a footnote, Roebuck (1977) claims further improvement when adrenaline 0.3 mg (0.3 ml of 1 in 1000 solution) is added to Dimer X.

Such comparisons are difficult to evaluate when compared with other centres, as significant technical variations are present; Hall (1974), for example, uses a contrast medium containing sodium. Each arthrographer must assess his own requirements of time, quality and cost. If cost is not important, certainly Dimer X and adrenaline seem to have no adverse qualities and will improve the results if any delay occurs.

The latest water-soluble medium to be used has been metrizamide ('Amipaque' Norgaard). Evidence from studies comparing metrizamide with meglumine-sodium-diatrizoate indicates that, like Dimer X, deterioration of contrast quality can be delayed by the use of this medium and that a lesser subsequent joint effusion is produced (Johansen *et al.*, 1977).

Both Dimer X and Amipaque, for different chemical reasons, have lower osmolalities than ionic monomer media and are consequently less likely to produce dilution or effusion, because of the reduced osmotic effect.

Financial considerations apart, it could be that metrizamide in an appropriate concentration, with or without adrenaline, is the best contrast medium. However, this medium, Amipaque, is so expensive at the present time that its use is quite unjustifiable to achieve only a marginal improvement in the quality of arthrographic detail.

1.5 Basic principles

Arthrography of the knee is not difficult, but requires considerable experience. Certain considerations have to be made in its performance.

1.5.1 Before performance of the examination

(a) The indications for the examination should be clear; a clinical diagnosis or impression must be sought, even if it is that no clinical diagnosis is possible. The clinician should draw the radiologist's attention to any specific problem. Such co-operation between the clinician and radiologist can only benefit the patient.

(b) The radiologist should take his own history, in addition to reading the referral note; the situation may have changed. A brief clinical examination of the knee without causing the patient any discomfort is highly desirable, both from the viewpoint of the diagnosis and in determining individual variation in structure of the knee.

(c) Recent plain films of the knee must be available or obtained prior to arthrography.

(d) The examination is performed in an X-ray department with well-maintained equipment, adequate for the purpose. Facilities for a satisfactory aseptic procedure must be present.

(e) The nature of the examination should be explained simply to the patient, including what he will feel and what the after-effects may be. This is the radiologist's responsibility: a very good chance exists that the clinician has told him only that he is being sent for a 'special X-ray', with no mention of needles. A history of allergy should be excluded.

1.5.2 Puncture of the joint

(a) Strict aseptic conditions are essential.

(b) Landmarks are identified with care before proceeding.

(c) Once in the joint the needle should not be advanced any further. The articular cartilage will be damaged and the patient caused discomfort.

(d) At each stage of injection of contrast medium, a check is made to ensure that the needle is still in a satisfactory intra-articular position.

(e) If doubt exists about the needle's position, stop and check. If necessary, fluoroscopic apparatus is used and observation made as a small amount of positive contrast medium is injected. Fortunately, the injection of quite large amounts of gas or medium outside the joint does not inconvenience the patient to a great degree. It is just unnecessary and careless.

(f) If the trainee arthrographer is really perplexed, a second opinion must be sought. This is a sign of strength, not weakness. If nobody is available to advise him, something is wrong with the way the department is run; perhaps it should not be undertaking such investigations.

1.5.3 Fluoroscopic procedure

(a) It is important to ensure that the patient is in the ideal position before bringing the apparatus into position across the table. It is so much more difficult afterwards.

(b) Fluoroscopy should be delayed until everything else is ready. The examination should begin with the diaphragms closed, then opened to the required size for spot films, not the other way round.

(c) A routine should be followed, modifying it if necessary, but not erratically moving from one end of the meniscus to the other. Consideration should be given to the assisting radiographer and those who may wish to interpret the films.

(d) Radiation dosage is limited by screening only when appropriate, by not repeating films of identical locations or views that are not orthograde or double contrast. In the latter circumstances, the reason should be sought (the traction band or the patient may have slipped down the table). The same approach applies to the need to expend excessive energy; arthrography does not require Herculean qualities.

(e) Neither haste nor lingering is appropriate. A clear understanding of the objectives makes for a quick, successful and diagnostic examination; as in most radiological procedures, however, no short-cut can take the place of experience.

References

Andrén, L. and Wehlin, L. (1960). Double contrast arthrography of knee with horizontal roentgen ray beam. *Acta Orthopaedica Scandinavica*, **29**, 307–14.

Bernstein, M.A. and Arens, R.A. (1926). Diagnostic inflation of the knee joint. *Radiology*, **7**, 500–6.

Bircher, E. and Oberholzer, J. (1934). Die Kniegelenkkapsel im Pneumoradiographiebild. *Acta Radiologica*, **15**, 452.

Burmann, M.S., Tumik, I.S. and Pomeranz, M. (1932).The injection of lipiodol into the knee joint. A warning against its use. *American Journal of Roentgenology*, **28**, 787.

Butt, W.P. and McIntyre, J.L. (1969). Double-contrast arthrography of the knee. *Radiology*, **92**, 487–99.

Cullen, C.H. and Chance, G.Q. (1943). Air arthrography in lesions of the semilunar cartilages. *British Journal of Surgery*, **30**, 241–5.

Freiberger, R.H., Killoran, P.J. and Cardona, G. (1966). Arthrography of the knee by double contrast method. *American Journal of Roentgenology*, **97**, 736–47.

Grech, P. (1977). *Hip arthrography*. Chapman & Hall, London.

Hall, F.M. (1974). Epinephrine enhanced knee arthrography. *Radiology*, **111**, 215–7.

Hoffa, A. (1906). Über Röntgenbilder nach Sauerstoffeinblasung in das Kniegelenk. *Berliner Klinische Wochenschrift*, **43**, 940–5.

Johansen, J.G., Lilleås, F.G. and Nordshus, T. (1977). Arthrography of the knee joints with Amipaque. *Acta Radiologica*, **18**, 523–8.

Johnson, R.J., Kettelkamp, D.B., Clark, W. and Leaverton, P. (1974). Factors affecting late results after meniscectomy. *Journal of Bone and Joint Surgery*, **56–A**, 719–29.

Lindblom, K. (1948). Arthrography of the knee joint. *Acta Radiologica (Stockholm) Supplement*, **74**.

Meschan, I and McGaw, W.H. (1947). Newer methods of pneumo-arthrography of the knee with evaluation of the procedure in 315 operated cases. *Radiology*, **49**, 675–710.

Rauenbusch, L. (1906). Zur Roentgendiagnoste der Meniskusverletzungen des Kniegelenkes. *Fortschritte auf dem Gebiele der Röntgenstrahlen*, **10**, 350–2.

Ricklin, P., Rüttiman, A. and Del Buono, M.S. (1971). *Meniscus Lesions. Practical Problems of Clinical Diagnosis, Arthrography and Therapy*. Georg Thieme, Verlag, Stuttgart.

Roebuck, E.J. (1977). Double contrast knee arthrography. Some new points of technique including the use of Dimer X. *Clinical Radiology*, **28**, 247–57.

Tapper, E.M. and Hoover, N.W. (1969). Late results after meniscectomy. *Journal of Bone and Joint Surgery*, **51–A**, 517–26.

Tegtmeyer, C.J., McCue, F.C., Higgins, S.M. and Ball, D.W. (1979). Arthrography of the knee: A comparative study of the accuracy of single and double contrast techniques. *Radiology*, **132**, 37–41.

Van der Berg, F. and Crèvecoeur, M. (1951). Etude anatomique et radiologique du genou arthrographie. *Journal Belge de Radiologie*, **34**, 7–82.

Werndorff, K.R. and Robinson, H. (1905). *Verhandlungen der deutschen Gesellschaft für orthopädische Chirurgie*, 4th Congress, pp. 9–10. Stuttgart: Verlag von Ferdinand Enke.

2 Anatomy of the knee joint

Any radiologist who wishes to understand meniscal disorders must possess a working knowledge of the anatomy and function of the knee joint, the most complicated joint in the body.

2.1 Bones forming the joint

The knee joint is formed by the distal end of the femur, the proximal end of the tibia and the patella. All the opposing surfaces are covered with articular cartilage. Three articulations are present – the patello-femoral joint and two tibio-femoral joints. However, both the synovial cavity and the articular surface of the femur are in continuity, although the latter is divided into tibial and patellar surfaces, two faint grooves, which cross the condyles obliquely forming the junction. The patellar surface is saddle-shaped and asymmetrical, with a larger lateral part accommodating the larger lateral surface of the patella. The tibial surfaces of the femur are separated by the intercondylar fossa into a medial surface which is longer, but narrower, than the surface of the lateral condyle. The articular surface of the lateral condyle sometimes shows a small central groove in the coronal plane.

The lateral condyle possesses a prominent epicondyle. The groove which lies between the epicondyle and the articular margin has a deepened anterior extremity, which gives attachment to the popliteus tendon. The posterior part of this groove accommodates the tendon only in full flexion of the knee. In extension, the tendon passes across the articular margin and sometimes indents it.

The tibia has two articular surfaces, a medial facet which is oval and slightly concave and a lateral facet which is more rounded. The two facets slope slightly towards each other and are separated by the roughened intercondylar area with its central intercondylar eminence bearing medial and lateral tubercles. The various structures attached to this surface are shown in Fig. 2.1. It is perhaps opportune to mention that, contrary to medical folklore, the anterior and posterior cruciate ligaments are not attached to the tips of these two tubercles and that bony fragments or ossicles, observed close to the tubercles on plain films, usually do not indicate previous cruciate avulsion injuries.

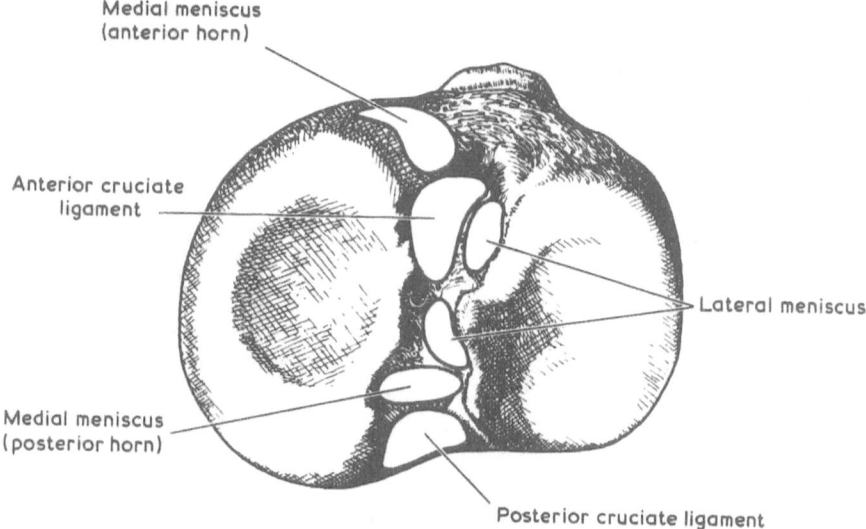

Fig. 2.1 *Diagram of the superior surface of the tibia* showing the attachments of the ligamentous and meniscal structures. Note that the posterior cruciate ligament is attached to the posterior margin of the tibia, whilst the anterior cruciate ligament attachment is not at the anterior margin but behind the attachment of the anterior horn of the medial meniscus. Neither ligament arises from a tibial spine. The diagram illustrates the discrepancy in size of the articular surfaces of the two tibial condyles.

The majority of the tibial articular surface is not in contact with the femur, but with the under surfaces of the menisci.

2.2 Synovial cavity

This is limited peripherally by the capsular attachments, but extends proximally from the patello-femoral articulation to form the large suprapatellar pouch. The synovial cavity can be divided into two compartments.

The *anterior* compartment lies in front of the tibio-femoral axis. It communicates with the suprapatellar pouch (Fig. 2.2), which often possesses an incomplete oblique septum (Fig. 2.3). Very rarely, the pouch is a completely separate bursa. The anterior compartment is encroached upon by the infrapatellar fat pad which occupies the space between the capsule, reinforced by the ligamentum patellae, and the synovium (Fig. 2.2). Synovial folds are to be found in relation to this and other fat pads.

The *posterior* compartment likewise is encroached upon by a posterior fat pad, which lies centrally and partially divides the compartment. A number of bursae connect with the posterior synovial space. Six postero-medial bursae are described

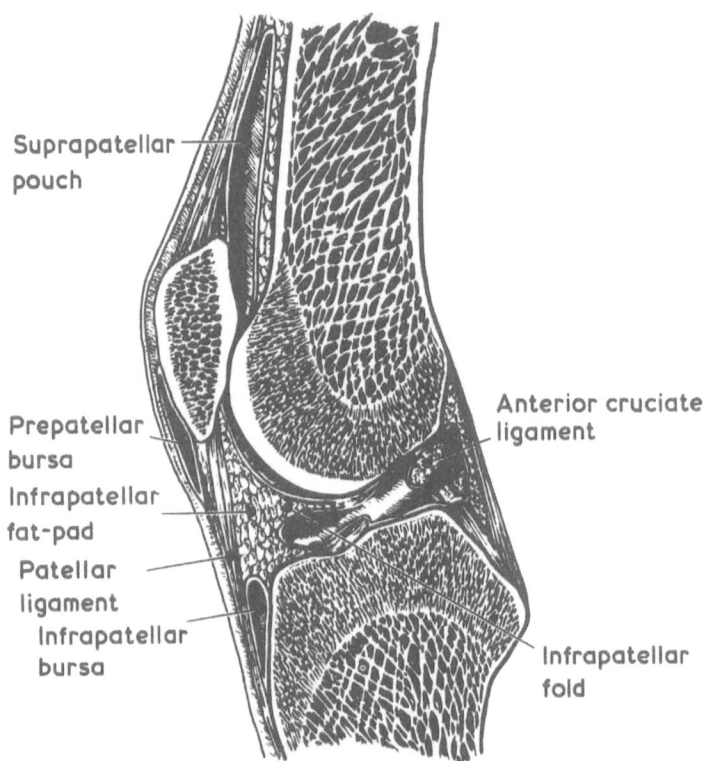

Fig. 2.2 *Sagittal cross-section of the knee joint* showing
the anatomical relationships. Several of the common
anterior bursae are shown. The infrapatellar fat-pad
and its relationship to the infrapatellar fold is
demonstrated, as is the synovial reflection over the
anterior cruciate. The suprapatellar pouch is shown to
communicate with the main synovial space at the
patello-femoral articulation. A layer of fat separates
the femoral cortex from the suprapatellar pouch.

(Wilson *et al.*, 1938), but these may combine and are mostly of little interest to the
radiologist.

The gastrocnemio-semimembranosus bursa is a fairly constant structure,
although occasionally it does not connect with the joint. More usually, it arises by a
narrow-necked opening on the medial side of the posterior compartment above the
level of the medial meniscus. It then expands to a variable degree into a sac, which
passes both between the medial head of gastrocnemius and the tendon of
semimembranosus (Fig. 2.4) and between the tendon of semimembranosus and the

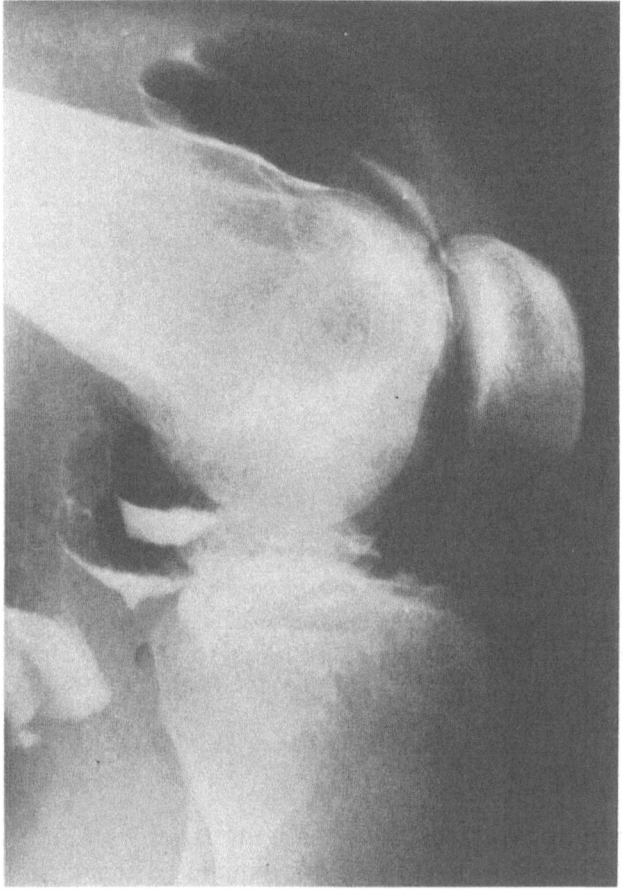

Fig. 2.3 *Lateral view of double contrast arthrogram.*
A septum crossing the suprapatellar pouch obliquely
causes an incomplete division of the bursa into two
parts. The infrapatellar fat pad is shown and a small
gastrocnemio-semimembranosus bursa is present in the
popliteal fossa.

capsule overlying the medial condyle of the femur, extending sometimes between
the tendons of semimembranosus and semitendinosus.

Occasionally, (a) only a small gastrocnemius bursa lies deep to its medial head,
or (b) a bursa is present between the semimembranosus tendon and the capsule
(Fig. 2.4).

Other bursae are occasionally observed at arthrography; on the lateral side of the
joint a bursa is rarely shown lying between the lateral head of gastrocnemius and
the joint capsule (Fig. 2.5).

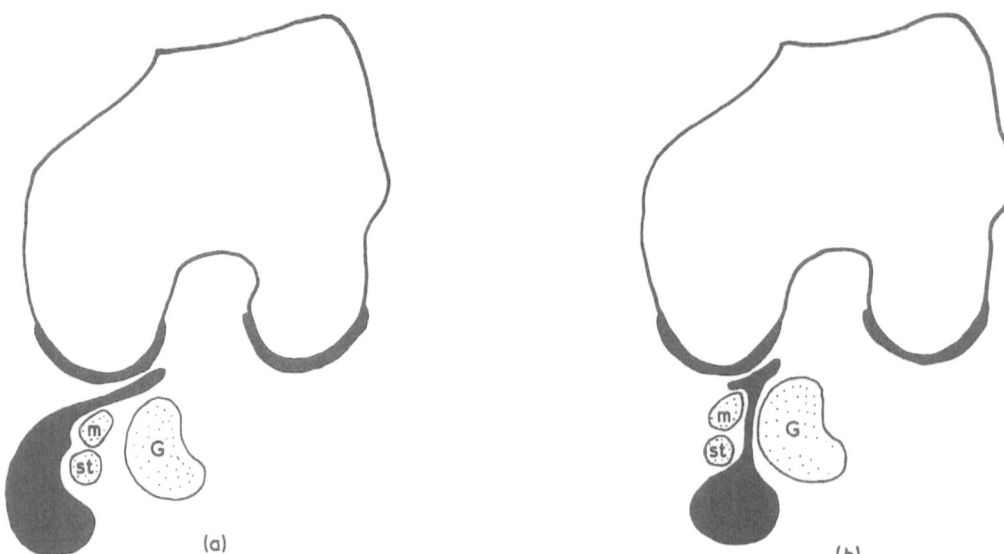

Fig. 2.4 *Diagram of gastrocnemio-semimembranosus bursal variants* (synovial space depicted in black). (a) The bursa has expanded and tracked medial to both the tendons of the semimembranosus (m) and the semitendinosus (st). (b) The bursa has passed between the semimembranosus and the medial head of the gastrocnemius (G).

The incidence of bursal communication with the knee joint varies with different studies and reflects the bias of surgical studies in symptomatic patients. Smillie (1970) quotes an incidence of communication of 50 per cent in normal knees between the gastrocnemio-semimembranosus bursa and the joint. Communication of *some* postero-medial bursae in arthrographic studies (presumably none are entirely normal knees) is higher than this figure, but most of such bursae are essentially normal in appearance.

The anterior and posterior compartments are divided incompletely into superior and inferior spaces by the menisci. The synovial reflection on the medial side of the inferior space is usually more or less at the tibial articular margin, whilst on the lateral side it may extend for several millimetres further down the lateral aspect of the tibia.

The suprapatellar pouch is a large communicating bursa extending proximally between the quadriceps muscle and tendon and the anterior surface of the femur (Fig. 2.2). It overlaps the femur slightly on both sides (Fig. 2.5). It is separated on both its superficial and deep surfaces from surrounding structures by adipose tissue, this prefemoral fat layer (Fig. 2.2) being of considerable thickness in some obese patients.

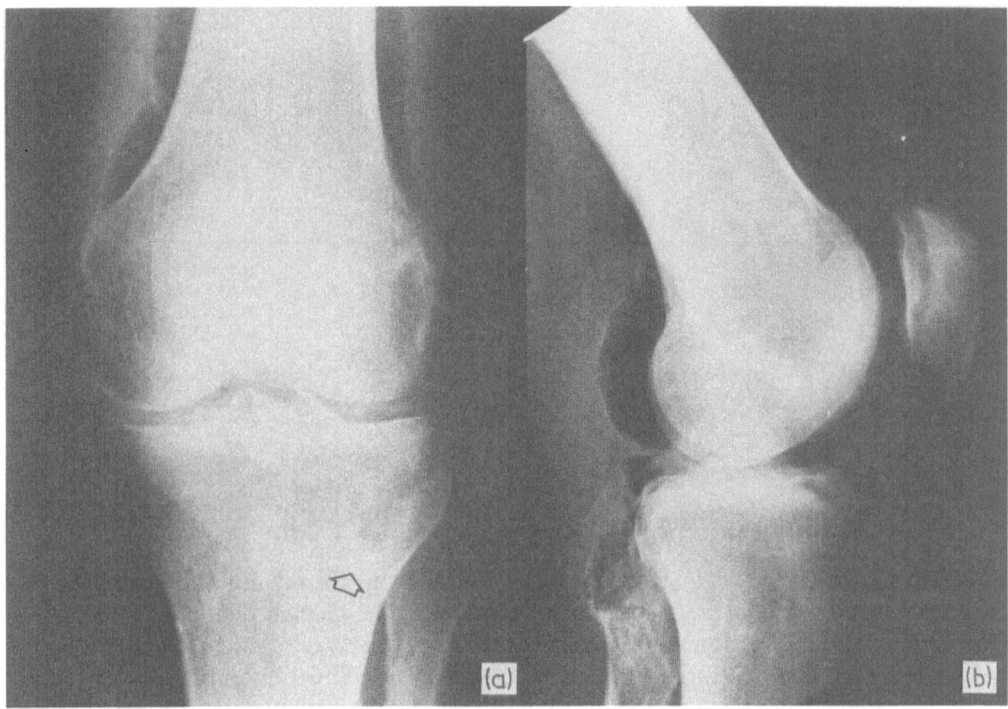

Fig. 2.5, (a) and (b) *Lateral bursa of the knee joint* between the capsule and the lateral head of the gastrocnemius muscle (arrow). The antero-posterior radiograph, (b), also illustrates how the distended suprapatellar pouch overlaps the femur, explaining how a large joint effusion may be visualized on the plain film.

2.3 Menisci

The menisci are fibrocartilage structures of wedge-shaped cross-section that serve to deepen the tibial articulation so that weight is distributed over a larger area. It is, in fact, suggested that incongruity of weight-bearing joints is the norm and that this is produced in the knee by the menisci (Goodfellow and O'Connor, 1975). Whether this is so or not, by deepening the joint they add to stability. Each meniscus has bony attachments for anterior end and posterior horns to the intercondylar area of the tibia (Fig. 2.1). The attachments of the lateral meniscus lie between those of the medial meniscus.

The *medial meniscus* (Fig. 2.6) is C-shaped and larger than the lateral. Its average width is 10mm, but its posterior horn is its widest part, and wider than any part of the lateral meniscus. Apart from its bony attachments to the tibia, its anterior horn is frequently connected with the insertion of the anterior cruciate ligament and the transverse ligament of the knee (Figs. 2.6 and 2.7) connects it with

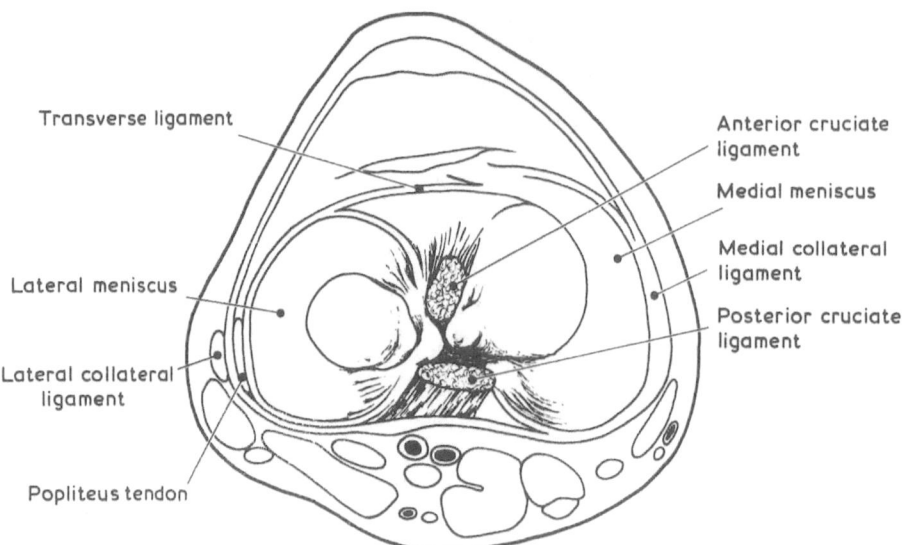

Fig. 2.6 *Cross-section at the level of the knee joint* showing the menisci and ligaments. Observe that the medial meniscus is firmly attached to the medial collateral ligament, whilst the popliteus tendon is interposed between the lateral collateral ligament and the lateral meniscus. The area of articular contact afforded by the menisci is demonstrated.

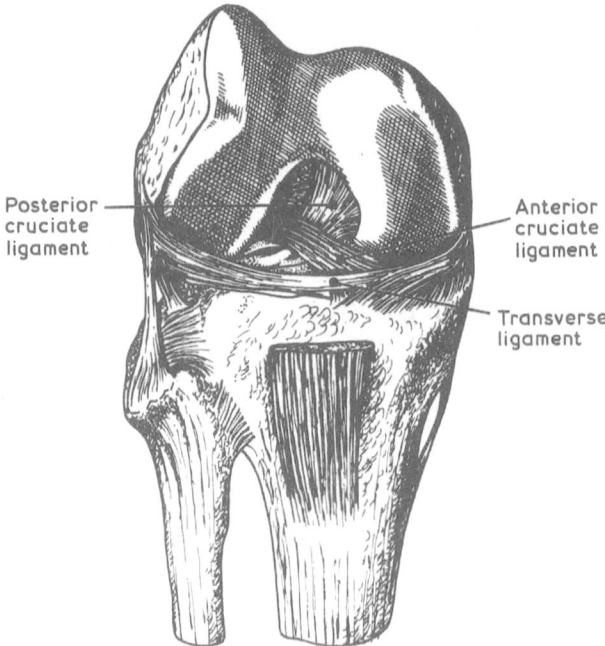

Fig. 2.7 *The knee joint dissected from the front* showing the transverse and cruciate ligaments.

the anterior margin of the lateral meniscus. Its posterior horn is firmly attached to the tibia whilst its peripheral fibres are fused with the capsule and the medial collateral ligament (Fig. 2.6), so that its mobility is strictly limited.

The *lateral meniscus* (Fig. 2.6) comprises a greater arc of a circle of smaller diameter and, although its average width is greater than the medial meniscus, its width is more uniform. Its shape is, however, variable. The anterior and posterior horns are firmly attached to the tibial intercondylar area. Fibres from the posterior horn pass superomedially to be attached to the medial femoral condyle. They divide at the lateral margin of the posterior cruciate ligament to form the anterior (Humphrey) and posterior (Wrisberg) menisco-femoral ligaments (Fig. 2.8).

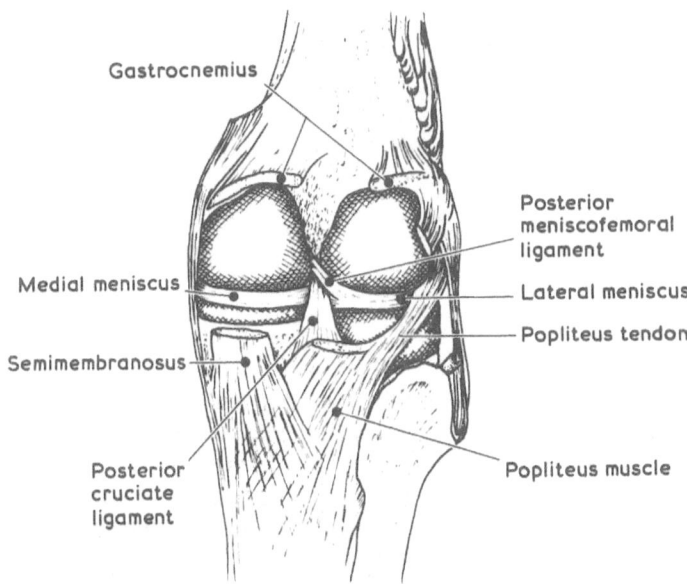

Fig. 2.8 *The knee joint dissected from behind.* The attachment of the posterior menisco-femoral ligament to the lateral meniscus is shown.

The lateral meniscus differs significantly from the medial by reason of its unique relationship with the tendon of the popliteus muscle. The popliteus has its origin (technically its *insertion*) from the posterior aspect of the proximal shaft of the tibia. Just below the level of the knee joint, it is inserted into a tendon which passes upwards and laterally to reach the capsule of the joint. The medial fibres of the tendon are inserted into the capsule and the posterior horn of the lateral meniscus (Last, 1948), whilst the main tendon passes deep to the capsule to gain its femoral insertion (Fig. 2.9). An important band of its fibres (previously described as the arcuate ligament) passes laterally to be attached to the head of the fibula.

By its course, the tendon is interposed between the postero-lateral part of the

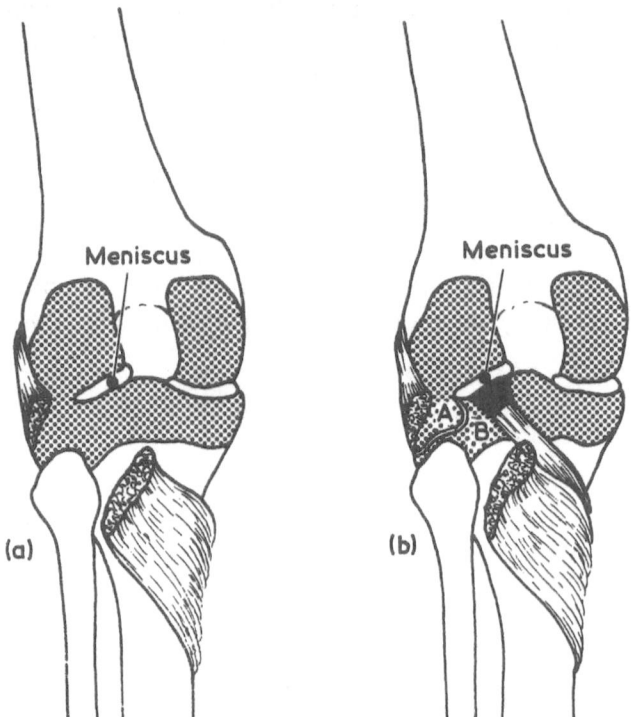

Fig. 2.9 *Diagram to show the femoral attachment of the popliteus tendon.*
(a) Traditional concept of the relationship of the tendon to the lateral meniscus,
showing the tendon passing into its sheath without direct attachment. (b) True
anatomical situation, as established by Last (1948). Although the superior (A) and
inferior (B) contributions of the synovial cavity are normally fused, they may be
separated occasionally, when a wider attachment of the popliteus tendon extends
across the whole posterior aspect of the meniscus.

meniscus and the lateral collateral ligament. It usually lies just beneath the
synovium lining a tendon sheath (the popliteus tendon sheath). This sheath passes
obliquely upwards and forwards with the tendon and separates it from the
meniscus, which is secured above and below by delicate attachments of fibrous
tissue covered on both surfaces by synovium. The popliteus tendon sheath,
therefore, has a floor and a roof bounded by the meniscal attachments. These,
however, are defective normally at two points: posteriorly, where the sheath
penetrates the inferior attachment and anteriorly, where the sheath penetrates the
superior attachment to become continuous with the synovial cavity proper in its
lateral expansion (Fig. 2.10).

It is only by understanding the anatomical arrangement that the radiologist can
evaluate the posterior horn of the lateral meniscus and determine whether

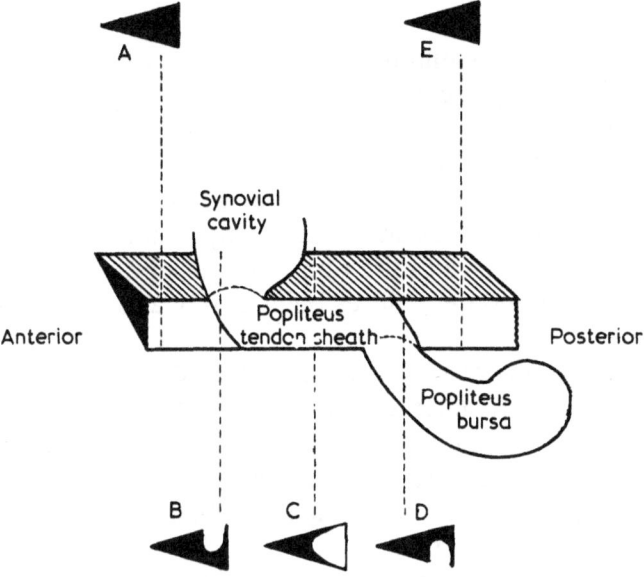

Fig. 2.10 *Diagram to show the relationship of the popliteus tendon sheath to the attachments of the lateral meniscus.* The diagram indicates how the arthrographic appearance produces defects in the peripheral attaching bands superiorly at B and inferiorly at D in the normal subject. At A and E, which are beyond the level of the tendon sheath, the meniscus is firmly attached peripherally. At C, both the peripheral attaching bands are intact.

peripheral detachment has occurred. The nomenclature of the peripheral attachments of the posterior lateral segment of the lateral meniscus is not generally approved. They are essentially suspensory ligaments and I shall refer to them as superior and inferior bands*.

The loose lateral attachment of the lateral meniscus means that its normal mobility is greater than that of the medial (Schaer, 1938).

2.4 Articular cartilage

The articular cartilage covers all joint surfaces. It measures some 3 to 4 mm in depth in the normal young adult and is nourished by the synovial fluid. No articular cartilage is present on the intercondylar area of the tibia or femur.

---

*The most general term used has been 'strut'. Jelaso (1975) has objected, I believe correctly, to this name on semantic grounds. His choice of 'fascicle' is no more acceptable, meaning a bundle of fibres, whilst these are ribbon-like bridges. Jelaso says 'we . . . call these small bands . . . fascicles'. Now why not call them by the short *Middle English* word 'band' ('a tape-like strand of tissue . . . connects other structures together' – Butterworths Medical Dictionary, 2nd Edition, 1978).

2.5 Ligaments

The knee joint is surrounded by a ligamentous capsule except where bursae, including the suprapatellar pouch, are present. Those parts of the capsule which attach the peripheral margins of the menisci to the tibia have been designated the coronary ligaments. The capsule is reinforced by the medial collateral ligament, a broad band of fibres. Anteriorly it blends with the patellar ligament. The outer fibres of the medial collateral ligament arise at and distal to the adductor magnus. Its distal attachment is to the medial surface of the tibia, superficial fibres passing below the level of the tibial tubercle and deep fibres being firmly attached to the medial meniscus (Fig. 2.6).

The lateral ligament of the knee is a cord-like structure separate from the lateral fibres of the capsule. Its extends from the lateral femoral epicondyle, just anterior to the popliteal groove, to the head of the fibula anterior to its most proximal point (Fig. 2.7), splitting the tendon of the biceps in so doing.

The cruciate ligaments are intra-articular, intra-capsular, but extra-synovial, structures, being invaginated into the synovial cavity from behind, so that a synovial covering is present on both sides, but anteriorly only on the anterior cruciate (Fig. 2.1).

The anterior cruciate ligament is attached to the intercondylar area of the tibia between the attachments of the anterior horns of the menisci and passes upwards and backwards to gain attachment to the medial aspect of the lateral femoral condyle (Fig. 2.7).

The posterior cruciate ligament is likewise attached to the tibia, but to the posterior margin of the intercondylar area. It passes forwards to be attached to the lateral surface of the medial femoral condyle (Fig. 2.7).

2.6 Movements of the knee joint

The knee is a hinge joint which also allows some rotary movement except in full extension. Maintenance of its integrity is a function of a combination of the bone structure of the tibia and femur, the surrounding muscles and tendons, the articular capsule and the intrinsic ligaments and cartilage.

In full extension, the knee is fixed by capsular and ligamentous structures, as well as by the 'screw home' movement of medial rotation which results from the provision of asymmetrical articular surfaces for the two femoral condyles (Fig. 2.7).

Flexion to 20° relaxes the collateral and cruciate ligaments because the femoral condyles decrease in size posteriorly. Minor relative collateral instability in incomplete extension is, therefore, physiological.

With flexion, rotatory movements are permitted, the femoral condyles gliding on those of the tibia. The axis of rotation is through the medial femoral condyle, so that greater displacement of the lateral femoral condyle occurs. Lateral and rotatory movement of the knee in flexion and extension is controlled by capsular, collateral and cruciate ligaments, except that in flexion the lateral ligament of the knee plays no part, being completely relaxed (Brantigan and Voshell, 1941). Forward gliding of the tibia on the femur ('anterior drawer' manoeuvre) is controlled by the anterior cruciate ligament and the thick posterior fibres of the lateral joint capsule. Backward gliding is controlled mainly by the posterior cruciate ligament. In this short section, a detailed description on bibliography of the unstable knee is neither possible nor necessary. The radiologist should be aware that excess gliding movements are commonly due to defects of the cruciate ligaments, whilst rotatory abnormalities often involve the collateral ligaments. Injuries of single ligaments occur, but lesions of several ligaments with or without meniscal damage are common. The menisci are not static in normal knee movements. Flexion causes them to slide (Schaer, 1938) posteriorly in relationship to the tibial plateau. Movement of the lateral meniscus is always greater because of its less firm attachment. When a rotatory element is added to flexion, the movement of the lateral meniscus is even greater.

It would not be right to leave this section without a reference to the action of the popliteus muscle. Under static conditions it acts as an internal rotator of the tibia on the femur (Basmajian and Lovejoy, 1971). Further electromyographic studies indicate that during the swing and stance phases of walking, it continues to maintain such internal rotation (Mann and Hagy, 1977).

Anatomical and other studies indicate that it causes posterior withdrawal of the lateral meniscus, thereby affording some protection against injury of this structure (Fig. 2.9). A review of the current thought on the anatomy and actions of the popliteus tendon has been provided by Harley (1977).

2.7 Vascular and nervous supply of menisci

The arterial blood supply for the knee is derived from branches of the popliteal artery. Space permits only discussion of the blood supply to the menisci.

The parameniscal region contains small arteries within its connective tissue stroma. Small vessels pass centrally into the outer one-third of the meniscus. The inner two-thirds of each meniscus is presumed to be dependent upon the synovial fluid for its nutrition. Such vessels as are present are in the deeper layers of the meniscus. It is on account of this blood supply that: (a) most meniscal tears never heal; (b) peripheral detachments may heal spontaneously; (c) peripheral detachments may be associated with haemarthrosis, unlike other complicated meniscal tears.

Nerve fibres can be traced into the peripheral attachments of the menisci. They tend to accompany the blood vessels (Gardner, 1948) and no evidence exists that they extend into the inner two-thirds of the meniscus.

References

Basmajian, J.V. and Lovejoy, J.F. (1971). Functions of the popliteal muscle in man. *Journal of Bone and Joint Surgery,* **53–A,** 557–62.

Brantigan, O.C. and Voshell, A.F. (1941). The mechanics of the ligaments and menisci of the knee joint. *Journal of Bone and Joint Surgery,* **23,** 44–66.

Gardner, E. (1948). The innervation of the knee joint. *Anatomical Record,* **101,** 109–30.

Goodfellow, J.W. and O'Connor, J. (1975). The transmission of loads through the hip and knee: a hypothesis on the aetiology of osteoarthritis. *Journal of Bone and Joint Surgery,* **57–B,** 400.

Harley, J.D. (1977). An anatomic-arthrographic study of the relationships of the lateral meniscus and the popliteus tendon. *American Journal of Roentgenology,* **128,** 181–7.

Jelaso, D.V. (1975). The fascicles of the lateral meniscus: an anatomic-arthrographic correlation. *Radiology,* **114,** 335–9.

Last, R.J. (1948). The popliteus muscle and the lateral meniscus. *Journal of Bone and Joint Surgery,* **32–B,** 93–9.

Mann, R.A. and Hagy, J.L. (1977). The popliteus muscle. *Journal of Bone and Joint Surgery,* **59–A,** 924–7.

Schaer, H. (1938). *Der Meniscusschaden.* G. Thieme, Leipzig.

Smillie, I.S. (1970). *Injuries of the Knee Joint,* 4th Edn. Livingstone, Edinburgh.

Wilson, P.D., Eyre-Brook, A.L. and Francis, J.D. (1938). A clinical and anatomical study of the semimembranosus bursa in relation to popliteal cyst. *Journal of Bone and Joint Surgery,* **20,** 963–84.

3 Clinico-pathological considerations: indications and contra-indications

3.1 Mechanism of production of injury to the meniscus

The causes of injury to the menisci are many. The vast majority result from indirect injury and classification of the forces involved is well-nigh impossible. The medial meniscus is damaged more often than the lateral, the ratio varying from 2.5:1 in a large general series (Smillie, 1970) to a much greater value in special groups, e.g. miners. On the whole, with greater care in the accuracy of diagnostic methods over the years, the ratio has fallen, suggesting either a change in the incidence or that lesions of the lateral meniscus have been underdiagnosed in the past.

Abnormal forces applied to the knee are flexion, extension, rotation, valgus and varus stress and compression. Because the knee joint is fixed in full extension, most injuries confined to the menisci occur with the knee in at least 20° of flexion.

Many tears of the menisci occur in field sports or athletics. A common mechanism applies for the typical longitudinal tear of the medial meniscus. The subject is bearing weight, often with the foot firmly fixed to the ground by shoes fitted with studs or spikes. At the same time, on the semi-flexed knee, the femur is rotated laterally on the tibia (a movement equivalent to medial rotation at the knee), causing the medial meniscus to be displaced posteriorly. Sudden extension at this time, including the 'screw home' element, increases the tension in the medial meniscus, which may tear longitudinally or be detached peripherally (Fig. 3.1). Although large bucket-handle tears may result from a single traumatic episode, often small or incomplete longitudinal tears constitute the initial lesions; these are increasingly vulnerable, lengthen with further trauma, and may ultimately become displaced. Symptomatically, this sequence shows as episodes of 'giving way' or pain leading to true 'locking' of the joint. This feature indicates displacement of the meniscal fragment and often, but not always, a bucket-handle tear (Figs. 3.1 and 3.2).

The lateral meniscus, being more mobile, tends to become trapped less easily and is less subject to stress because of its loose peripheral attachment. For the same reasons, locking is less common.

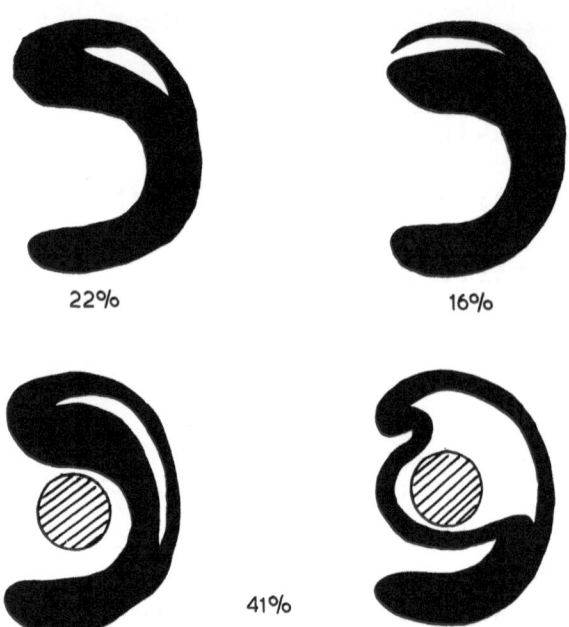

22%   16%

41%

Fig. 3.1 *Incidence of tears of posterior portion of medial meniscus* (Trillat, 1962). This diagram also shows the nature of displacement of a bucket-handle tear. The hatched area represents the area of contact of the femoral and tibial condyles.

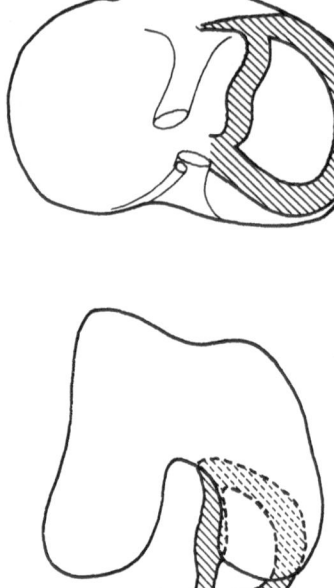

Fig. 3.2 *Bucket-handle tear of medial meniscus* demonstrating the central displacement of the incompletely detached rim of the meniscus and its relationship to the medial femoral condyle. Such a tear may become detached at either extremity, in due course, following further injury.

Degenerative changes in fibro-cartilage becomes apparent in the third and perhaps even the second decade of life. After the age of 30 years, histological changes are present in the meniscus, which must reduce its elasticity and resistance to stress. It is perhaps for this reason that, increasingly, after this age the nature of the injury may be more trivial, e.g. getting up awkwardly from a chair, and the character of the meniscal tear varies; horizontal ('cleavage', 'degenerative') tears are found. Smillie (1970) suggests that the changes of ageing produce rigidity and thinning of the articular cartilage, so that adduction and rotatory stress takes place within the meniscus itself and results in a horizontal tear (Fig. 3.3).

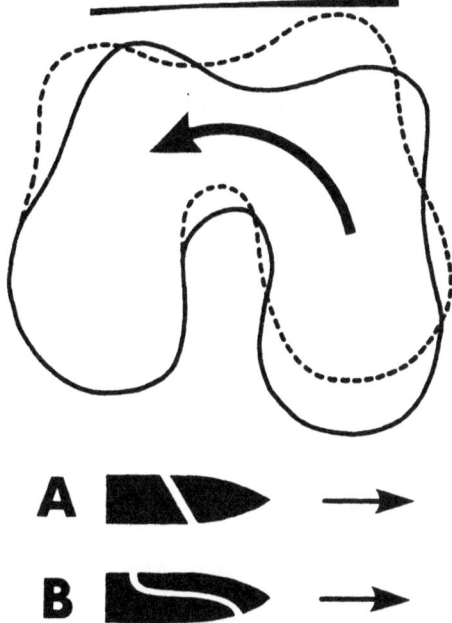

Fig. 3.3 *Vertical and horizontal tears of medial meniscus* (after Smillie, 1970). Diagram to indicate that whilst the same rotatory movement of the femur on the tibia is occurring in the weight-bearing knee, different types of tear may result. A – a vertical tear following injury in the young adult. B – a horizontal ('cleavage') tear occurring in the more degenerate meniscus of an older patient.

Prolonged work in a kneeling and, particularly, a squatting position, e.g. in miners, carpet-layers and dedicated kindergarten teachers, tends to produce damage to the posterior horn of the medial meniscus. This direct pressure on one part of the meniscus may accelerate the degenerative process, but also causes direct damage, with fibrillation, to both the femoral and tibial surfaces of the meniscus. Horizontal tears often develop an oblique extension to one or both meniscal surfaces, forming a flap which can, on occasions, produce intermittent or atypical locking.

The only merit of classification is convenience (Smillie, 1970). The tears sustained by the menisci rarely follow a simple linear pattern and, therefore, it is not always possible to classify them satisfactorily. The best one can hope for is to record the major direction of the tear, its extent and whether it is complete or incomplete. Many of the words used in surgical pathology are ambiguous. In relation to a C-shaped structure, such as a meniscus, such words as longitudinal, though accepted by long usage, have no specific meaning. If the term 'horizontal' is used for a cleavage tear, then perhaps 'vertical' should be employed for the tear perpendicular to it. (Clearly there could come a mid-point where 'oblique' would be more applicable, but this rarely poses a problem in practice). Only one further major direction in which a tear can occur is then left. Ricklin *et al.*(1971) refer to this as a transverse tear, but I prefer the term *radial,* which leads to less ambiguity. The primary directions in which a tear can occur are illustrated in Fig. 3.4.

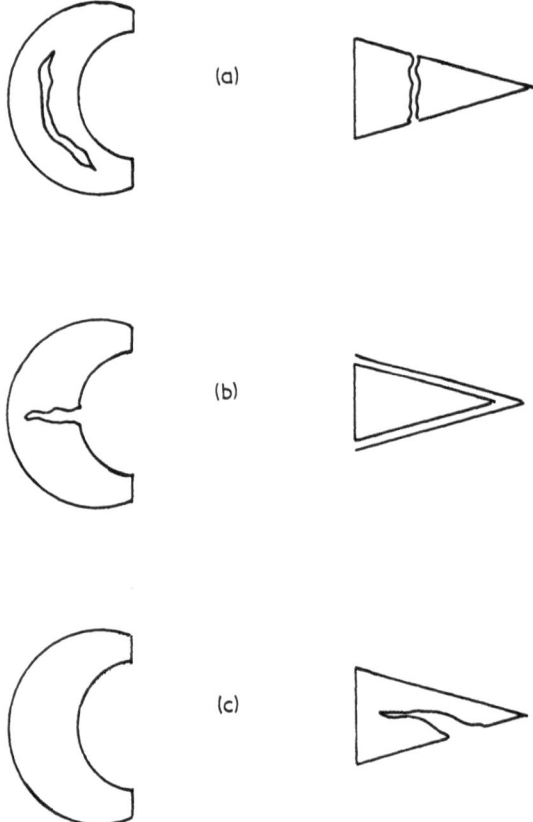

Fig. 3.4 *Meniscal tears: the three primary directions.* (a) Vertical (longitudinal). (b) Radial; the cross-sectional appearance varies and has been represented as incomplete superimposition of the two margins of the tear. (c) Horizontal; the tear in this instance is not visible from the superior surface.

Whilst it is not desirable to subdivide tears into smaller and smaller groups, it is worth mentioning one variety of tear, which characteristically affects the middle third of the lateral meniscus. This probably begins as a horizontal double cleavage tear (Smillie, 1970). Weakness of the unsupported free margin leads here to an additional radial tear, the final result being a curved tear of the free margin of the meniscus which those, with more imagination than ornithological expertise, have called a 'parrot-beak' tear.

The 'bucket-handle' tear is, however, well-named, as the term describes its appearance (an extensive vertical tear) and its behaviour (central displacement of the handle) (Fig. 3.2).

Tears of the menisci are often complicated by damage to the collateral ligaments, although the latter may heal before the patient presents clinically. Valgus strain, usually the result of a heavy blow to the lateral aspect of the knee, may rupture the medial collateral ligament. Continuation of the valgus stress will damage the attachments of the medial meniscus and the anterior cruciate ligament – the 'unhappy triad' (O'Donoghue, 1950).

Tenderness is usually present above and/or below the joint line at the ligamentous attachments. Isolated rupture of the lateral collateral ligament is uncommon. The cord-like ligament is less subject to rotatory stress and sufficient varus stress is usually found only in severe dislocating injuries.

The anterior cruciate ligament may rupture in isolation (Wang et al., 1975; McDaniel 1976), but is more often associated with medial collateral ligament and/or medial meniscus tears. Such associated injuries sometimes relate to the severity of the causative injury; fibres of the anterior cruciate ligament are frequently attached to the anterior horn of the medial meniscus, so that damage to this structure can be associated with a torn anterior cruciate ligament. Its intracapsular situation and its blood supply often result in haemarthrosis when it is torn acutely. An isolated tear of the anterior cruciate ligament produces little abnormal movement (Trickey et al., 1976); the presence of excessive tibio-femoral movement often indicates additional damage to the posterolateral fibres of the capsule with an anteromedial rotatory movement on pulling the tibia forward. Some authors (Hughston et al., 1976) believe that a torn anterior cruciate ligament is not the cause of an anterior drawer sign. They produce evidence to indicate that a tear of this ligament merely augments a capsular tear, usually menisco-tibial fibres, and they stress that the anterior drawer sign should always be elicited with the leg in both internal and external rotation. They found, under general anaesthesia, a positive anterior drawer sign in 77 per cent of patients with an intact anterior cruciate ligament.

The presence of a torn or lax anterior cruciate ligament suggests instability of the joint and sometimes a secondary associated medial meniscus injury. However, good quadriceps development can mask any deficiency due to such a rupture and produce a symptom-free knee.

Posterior cruciate ligament tears are less uncommon than previously supposed, especially in association with other ligamentous injuries (Trickey, 1968). Rupture results from forceful posterior displacement of the tibia with the knee flexed. The patient complains of the knee giving way backwards, and backward sagging of the tibia is apparent in the slightly flexed supine knee. A positive posterior drawer sign may be expected.

3.2 Diagnosis of internal derangement of the knee

It is not the intention to recount or discuss the clinical diagnosis of knee injuries. This subject is described in a number of standard works (Smillie, 1970; Ricklin *et al.*, 1971). It is necessary, however, to understand the basis of the clinical signs and their limitations, so that the use of arthrography and other diagnostic procedures can be put in perspective. The primary problem stems from the fact that diagnosis of a significant meniscal tear leads to meniscectomy. Meniscectomy, although one of the most common orthopaedic operations, is not a benign procedure (Huckell, 1965). Most short-term studies (Lipscomb and Henderson, 1947; Wynn Parry *et al.*, 1958; Nicholas *et al.*, 1970;) indicate relatively normal function of the knee in over three-quarters of patients after meniscectomy. A danger, therefore, exists that both surgeons and the public will regard meniscectomy as a harmless procedure with a generally excellent outcome. Long-term studies present a different picture. In groups reviewed approximately 10 years following meniscectomy, only about 40 per cent of patients are found to have normal knees (Huckell, 1965; Tapper and Hoover, 1969), although as many as 68 per cent could be classed as satisfactory clinical results. Johnson *et al.* (1974), but not Tapper and Hoover (1969), found that the longer the duration of symptoms and greater the frequency of re-injury before meniscetomy, the worse the final result.

As unqualified statements, these exaggerate the case, but perhaps no more so than the earlier over-optimistic forecasts of the value of meniscectomy. No controlled trial of patients with painful locking knees due to bucket-handle tears of a meniscus would be possible; undoubtedly such patients are improved by surgery, which corrects the immediate disability. Neither can a follow-up series of patients undergoing meniscectomy be expected where the meniscus was found to be entirely normal after removal!

What these and other studies do indicate, however, is that a meniscus should be removed only when it is definitely abnormal (Johnson *et al.*, 1974) and probably that the sooner its removal, after a definite tear, the better. This places a premium on accurate diagnosis.

In clinical diagnosis, although a confident diagnosis of a specific meniscal tear can be made in some patients, in a large proportion of cases a complicated diagnostic problem exists which can be solved only by balancing every shred of evidence which is available (Smillie, 1970).

Although often suggestive, the mechanism of injury coupled with the symptoms, does not usually establish the diagnosis. A history of true locking, however, is almost pathognomonic of a torn meniscus. A variety of clinical signs, mostly eponymous, are described, which relate to the ability to produce a snap or clunk by rotating the knee in flexion. Only when such snaps are due to a meniscal lesion is the test positive and only a lesion that will displace, i.e. a large posterior vertical tear, will produce the diagnostic snap. Thus, neither the presence nor absence of a positive McMurray's sign should be overemphasized. It is, after all, just a clinical sign and not to be considered in isolation.

Even after over 110 years of meniscectomy (Brodhurst, 1867), the overall accuracy of clinical diagnosis is unknown. This must be, to some extent, due to the difficulty of obtaining objective figures, the inability to visualize the whole structure at arthrotomy and, even after meniscectomy, the inability to confirm or exclude certain lesions, e.g. peripheral vertical tears or detachments, from inspection of the excised specimen. Accuracy in clinical diagnosis varies considerably, in part because the diagnosis of an internal derangement of the knee, or the need for an exploratory operation, has, in certain series, been equated with a correct diagnosis. Stewart (1971) states 'one is astute who can keep his errors in diagnosing tears as low as ten per cent'. In Smillie's (1970) figures of 8000 meniscectomies, only 4 per cent were without obvious pathology, giving an accuracy in management of 96 per cent. Similarly, Wynn Parry et al. (1958) reported only 6.2 per cent of menisci removed were normal (a further 4 per cent being intact, but hypermobile).

Accurate clinical diagnosis must depend upon the experience of the examiner and even in specialized teaching centres a clinical accuracy of 95 per cent or more cannot be expected when results are assessed objectively. Thus Nicholas et al. (1970) recorded an 80 per cent accuracy in clinical diagnosis, Bedford et al. (1979) 72.5 per cent and Jackson and Abe (1972) 68.5 per cent accuracy in a series of 'problem' knees.

If the accuracy of clinical diagnosis is not always acceptable, then ancillary methods of diagnosis will be sought. At the present time, in the diagnosis of internal derangements of the knee, to all practical purposes the choice of investigation lies between arthrography and arthroscopy. Other investigations which could have a place in future diagnostic techniques include CT scanning and transmitted ultrasonography; these are investigations neither developed in this field, nor readily available outside special centres in the United Kingdom.

3.2.1 Arthroscopy

Like arthrography, this is not a new investigation. Bircher (1921)first employed the Jacobaeus laparoscope for this purpose; this must have been a hazardous procedure as the bulb was free within the joint cavity, which he distended with gas. Modern arthroscopy began with the production of the Watanabe arthroscope and the publication of detailed illustrations of arthroscopic findings (Watanabe et al., 1957,

1968). More recently, instruments have been designed of narrower diameter and fitted with fibre-light optics.

Arthroscopy is a method of visualizing the intra-synovial structures without a formal arthrotomy, its only alternative. It has the advantage that the surgeon who proposes to operate, if such an operation proves necessary, personally sees the synovial cavity. It is possible to assess the state of the synovium itself and to determine whether inflammation is present. Meniscal tears can be identified, as can lesions of the articular cartilage, such as chondromalacia patellae, or the osteochondral juction, such as traumatic dissecting lesions (osteochondritis dissecans). The cruciate ligaments are visible by this technique, as are other synovial lesions, e.g. adhesions and intra-articular loose bodies. With this potential, it might be thought that arthroscopy denies the need for arthrography and, indeed, some arthroscopists believe this to be the case. Arthroscopy, however, possesses both defects and limitations. It is a service expensive in both time and equipment. The modern arthroscope and fittings can cost as much as £1500 and the procedure is performed in the operating theatre, limiting its use for therapeutic surgery. Ordinarily, general anaesthesia is administered, only a minority of surgeons being prepared to use local anaesthesia; this is because general anaesthesia permits a preliminary clinical examination with the patient completely relaxed and, during arthroscopy, a fuller visualization of all compartments is obtained (Bedford *et al.*, 1979). The need for general anaesthesia necessitates a stay in hospital, even if only as a day case. This, plus the services of surgeon, anaesthetist and theatre staff, makes arthroscopy a greater drain on hospital resources than arthrography. Some surgeons find it impossible to accept the opinion of a radiologist about the state of the menisci, whilst others now accept that arthrography provides valuable information to the team that is caring for the patient (of which the radiologist is a member).

The next point to be considered is the relative positions of the two investigations. Often, no choice presents itself; one or other investigation may not be available to the orthopaedic surgeon. In some other respects, the techniques are not in competition, but are complementary. Arthrography does not provide adequate information about the state of the synovium in most cases; it is less valuable in lesions of the articular cartilage and ligaments than is arthroscopy. The proponents of both investigations, however, usually claim that one method is the one of choice for demonstration of meniscal lesions. Both have their advantages and disadvantages. Arthroscopy requires experience to achieve technical accuracy, as does arthrography (De Haven and Collins, 1975), particularly in the interpretation of the spot-films. Arthroscopy fails to visualize directly the posterior horn of the meniscus and, although an indication of hypermobility or detachment may be obtained by external application of the examining finger or a probing needle, such indirect evidence is less than satisfactory and can be misinterpreted (Bedford *et al.*, 1979).

Arthroscopy cannot demonstrate horizontal tears of the under surface of the meniscus or the extent of cleavage tears within the meniscal substance. Too many arthroscopists regard arthrography as a static procedure, with the serial X-ray films as the sole outcome of the examination. This is equivalent to considering coloured photographs taken at arthroscopy as the only end-result. Both examinations are, of course, dynamic – the meniscus being visualized under stressing movements of the knee – only differing in the type of anaesthesia employed. When confined to meniscal lesions, arthrography has a high degree of accuracy (Freiberger *et al.*, 1966), less on the lateral than the medial side (Dalinka *et al.*, 1973), this being due principally to difficulty in the evaluation of peripheral detachments or partial detachments of the posterior horn of the lateral meniscus.

The accuracy of arthrography and arthroscopy in experienced hands is comparable; both investigations can be expected to achieve an accuracy of 85 to 95 per cent in the diagnosis of meniscal lesions. Unfortunately, it seems difficult to produce an unbiased series where the proponents of each investigation are of equivalent experience. Thus, in arthroscopic series (Jackson and Abe, 1972; De Haven and Collins, 1975), figures for the accuracy of an experienced arthroscopist are compared with arthrographic results which are admitted to be below those reported elsewhere in the literature. In a study confined to 'problem knees', undertaken at the Royal National Orthopaedic Hospital, both procedures gave an accuracy of 86 per cent. When the results of both procedures were taken together,

Table 3.1

	Arthrography	Arthroscopy
Performed by	Radiologist	Orthopaedic surgeon
Performed in	Radiology department	Operating theatre
Additional expensive equipment	None	Arthroscope
Experience required in (a) technique (b) interpretation	Yes Yes	Yes Yes
Anaesthetic	Usually local, sometimes none	Usually general, sometimes local
Main area of advantage	Meniscal tears	Articular and synovial surfaces
Main area of limitation	Articular and synovial surfaces	Posterior horn tears of menisci
Overall accuracy in experienced hands	Excellent	Excellent

the diagnostic accuracy rose to 98 per cent, indicating that the nature of the errors was different in the two procedures (Ireland *et al.*, 1980).

In Table 3.1, the differences between the two diagnostic methods have been recorded. No attempt has been made to denote whether any point favours a particular investigation. The fact that a radiologist performs arthrography may be an adverse factor to a surgeon who is unwilling to delegate any part of the pre-operative investigation and a boon to the surgeon who is short of time, beds or operating sessions.

In the fortunate centre where both arthrography and arthroscopy are freely available, it is clearly possible to develop a plan of action where, if an investigatory procedure is required, the one most likely to provide a clear answer to the clinical problem should be employed. Thus, if an isolated tear of the anterior cruciate ligament is thought to be present, arthroscopy might precede operation; if an undisplaced tear of the posterior horn of the medial meniscus is suspected, then arthrography is a better primary investigation. If both investigations are performed within a short period, arthrography should precede arthroscopy; in the week following arthroscopy, due to leakage from the synovial cavity and joint effusion, a high-quality arthrogram is not usually achieved.

3.2.2 Knee arthrography

3.2.2.1 Indication and contraindications

The indication for arthrography can be simplified by designating its value in the 'problem knee' or in investigation of any internal derangement where the diagnosis is in doubt, particularly the presence or absence of a meniscal lesion. A fuller list of indications is suggested in Table 3.2.

Table 3.2 Indication for knee arthrography

---

1. Acute injuries, especially in athletes and breadwinners, where a premium exists in initiating effective treatment.
2. Whenever a discrepancy exists between symptoms and clinical signs, or low-grade symptoms persist.
3. Where, as a result of varying symptoms and signs, although a meniscus injury is suspected, the side affected cannot be localized.
4. In injuries, thought to be minor, which do not respond to treatment.
5. Recurrent or persistent joint effusions.
6. Locked knees (sometimes), prior to unlocking.
7. Prior to major repair or reconstructioin of ligaments, to exclude a meniscus injury.
8. In the case of persistent complaints following meniscectomy.
9. In all children where a meniscus lesion is diagnosed clinically.
10. For documentation in disability and compensation cases.
11. In the differential diagnosis of deep vein thrombosis and large or ruptured popliteal cysts.
12. In a variety of other disorders, with a variable return of diagnostic information (see Chapter 8).

Absolute contraindications comprise only a generalized infective illness, the presence of local infection in the region of the knee, or a clear history of allergy. Modification of the technique to gas arthrography alone, on the basis of a strong allergic history, has been required on only two occasions in our first 1000 cases. No allergic manifestations have been observed in our patients undergoing arthrography and perhaps even in these two patients we were overcautious. The absence of allergic response probably results from: (1) small amount of iodine-containing contrast medium injected; (2) injection into synovial cavity.

Relative contraindications include bleeding diseases, acute or chronic synovitis, where the return on the examination would be greatly increased by allowing the inflammation to settle, and gross degenerative change on the plain films, where little information is to be gained except, perhaps, in the demonstration of loose bodies. In such patients fragmented menisci may be expected.

3.2.2.2 Complications

Few complications are observed in arthrography. Following the completion of the examination, the patient will be aware of some excess gas and fluid in the knee; this rarely causes any disability. Very rarely, in the 12 hours or so following arthrography, an *effusion* of significant size may arise and become tense and painful. Aspiration may be required for symptomatic relief and the fluid should then be sent for bacteriological examination. Such a synovitis is probably chemical in nature.

Production of a *septic arthritis* has been reported on rare occasions but should not occur and indicates some flaw in the aseptic technique. No such complication has been observed in our series. Even mild *allergic reactions* are infrequently observed at arthrography due to the small amount of iodine-containing medium injected into the joint, even in the presence of a history of reactions to intravenous media. A significant history of severe allergic reaction in the past necessitates the employment of the less diagnostic technique using only gas as the contrast agent.

References

Bedford, A., Aichroth, P. and Hutton, P. (1979). Arthroscopy: The first hundred are the worst. *Journal of the Royal Society of Medicine,* **72**, 6–12.

Bircher, E. (1921). Die Arthroendoskopie. *Zentralblatt für Chirurgie,* **48**, 1460–1.

Brodhurst, B.E. (1867). On loose cartilages in the joint. *St George's Hospital Reports,* **2**, 141–4.

Dalinka, M.K., Coren, G.S. and Wershba, M. (1973). Knee arthrography. *Critical Reviews in Clinical Radiology and Nuclear Medicine,* **4**, 1–59.

De Haven, K.E. and Collins, H.R. (1975). Diagnosis of internal derangements of the knee. The role of arthroscopy. *Journal of Bone and Joint Surgery,* **57-A**, 802–10.

Freiberger, R.H., Killoran, P.J. and Cardona, G. (1966). Arthrography of the knee by double contrast method. *American Journal of Roentgenology,* **97**, 736–47.

Huckell, JR. (1965). Is meniscectomy a benign procedure? A long term follow-up study. *Canadian Journal of Surgery*, **8**, 254–60.

Hughston, J.C., Andrews, J.R., Cross, M.J. and Moschi, A. (1976). Classification of knee ligament instabilities. Part I. The medial compartment and cruciate ligaments. *Journal of Bone and Joint Surgery*, **58–A**, 159–72.

Ireland, J., Trickey, E.L. and Stoker, D.J. (1980). Arthroscopy and arthrography of the knee: a critical review. *Journal of Bone and Joint Surgery*, **62–B**, 3–6.

Jackson, R.W. and Abe, I. (1972). The role of arthroscopy in the management of disorders of the knee – an analysis of 200 consecutive examinations. *Journal of Bone and Joint Surgery*, **54–B**, 310.

Johnson, R.J., Kettelkamp, D.B., Clark W. and Leaverton, R. (1974). Factors affecting late results after meniscectomy. *Journal of Bone and Joint Surgery*, **56–A**, 719–29.

Lipscomb, P.R. and Henderson, M.S. (1947). Internal derangements of the knee. *Journal of the American Medical Association*, **135**, 827–31.

McDaniel, W.J. (1976). Isolated partial tear of the anterior cruciate ligament. *Clinical Orthopedics*, **115**, 209–12.

Nicholas, J.A., Freiberger, R.H. and Killoran, P.J. (1970). Double-contrast arthrography of the knee. Its value in the management of 225 knee derangements. *Journal of Bone and Joint Surgery*, **52–A**, 203–20.

O'Donoghue, D.H. (1950). Surgical treatment of fresh injuries to the major ligaments of the knee. *Journal of Bone and Joint Surgery*, **32–A**, 721–38.

Ricklin, P., Rüttimann, A. and Del Buono, M.S. (1971). *Meniscus Lesions*. Georg Thieme Verlag, Stuttgart.

Smillie, I.S. (1970). *Injuries of the Knee Joint*, 4th Edn. Livingstone, Edinburgh.

Stewart, M. (1971). In: *Campbell's Operative Orthopaedics*, 5th edition (Crenshaw, A.H., ed), p. 909, The C.V. Mosby Co., St. Louis.

Tapper, E.M. and Hoover, N.W. (1969). Late results after meniscectomy. *Journal of Bone and Joint Surgery*, **51–A**, 517–26.

Trickey, E.L. (1968). Rupture of the posterior cruciate ligament of the knee. *Journal of Bone and Joint Surgery*, **50–B**, 334–41.

Trickey, E.L. (1976). Ligamentous injuries around the knee. *British Medical Journal*, **2**, 1492–4.

Trillat, A. (1962). Lésions traumatiques du ménisque interne du genou. Classement anatomique et diagnostic clinique. *Revue de Clinique Orthopédique*, **48**, 551–60.

Wang, J.B., Rubin, R.M. and Marshall, J.L. (1975). A mechanism of isolated anterior cruciate ligament rupture. *Journal of Bone and Joint Surgery*, **57–A**, 411–13.

Watanabe, M., Takeda, S. and Ikeuchi, H. (1957). *Atlas of Arthroscopy*. Igaku Shoin, Tokyo.

Watanabe, M., Takeda, S. and Ikeuchi, H. (1968). *Atlas of Arthroscopy*, 2nd Edn. Igaku Shoin, Tokyo.

Wynn Parry, C.B., Nichols, P.J.R. and Lewis, N.R. (1958). Meniscectomy: A review of 1723 cases. *Annals of Physical Medicine*, **4**, 201–15.

4 Technique

'There are more ways to the wood than one' *Old English Proverb*

Techniques evolve and local conditions vary, so it would be arrogant to suggest that only one correct way to perform arthrography exists. However, the practice of knee arthrography by a double-contrast fluoroscopic technique does entail the application of certain principles, without which the road can be hard and interminable. In this section, therefore, a technique is described and, where possible, why it is employed, stressing which features are essential, desirable or optional.

4.1 Joint puncture

After reassurance, explanation of the technique to be followed and taking a history, including one of allergy, the patient lies on the X-ray table where the radiologist briefly examines the knee clinically and confirms which side is to be examined radiologically. The patient lies supine with this knee to the accessible side of the table; his knee is supported on a 4½ in. (11.5 cm) high foam wedge so that it is relaxed, in slight flexion (Fig. 4.1). A sterile gown is unnecessary. A face mask is not essential , but can be an indication to all the staff that an aseptic techique is being performed. The contents of the arthrographic tray or pack are listed in Table 4.1. The skin of the knee is prepared using aseptic precautions; an iodine solution is favoured because (i) it is a most effective antiseptic agent, and (ii) its colouration reminds the radiologist at fluoroscopy later which knee is being examined, even under diminished lighting. Both the front and the sides of the knee are prepared aseptically as, at a later stage, it is necessary to hold the patella. It is generally easier to puncture the joint whilst facing the patient's head or feet, so if right-handed and performing arthrography on the right knee, the radiologist should stand beside the table facing caudally (this procedure is reversed for the other knee or if the arthrographer is left-handed). The patella is taken in the left hand and drawn laterally with the fingers whilst pressing firmly into the patello-femoral space

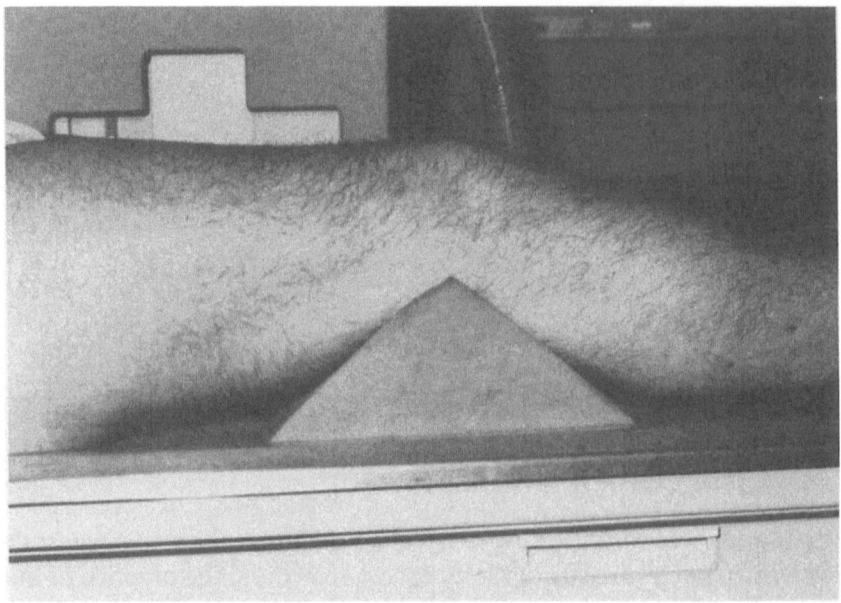

Fig. 4.1 Prior to puncture of the joint, the patient's knee is supported by a soft pad in slight flexion.

Table 4.1

Arthrographic tray	
Syringes (disposable)	1 20 ml
	1 10 ml
	1 5 ml
Needles	1 18 or 19 gauge 1½ in. needle
	(e.g. Gillette cream – ideally thin-wall, short bevel)
	1 25 gauge ⅝ in. needle (Gillette blue)
	1 three-way disposable plastic stopcock
	1 plastic connecting tube, e.g. roentgenography set (Becton–Dickinson)
	1 Kwill plastic filler tube or large-bore drawing-up needle
	Cotton balls and gauze squares
	1 sponge-holding forceps
	Dressing towel with 10 cm central hole
Other equipment	Sterile disposable gloves
	Conray 280 in ampoules
	Lignocaine 1% 2 ml or 5 ml ampoules
	Iodine solution or Betanidine for skin preparation
	CO_2 cylinder with regulator and tubing leading to gas stopcock and connecting with reservoir (disposable urine bag)
	Large artery forceps to seal efferent tube from reservoir.

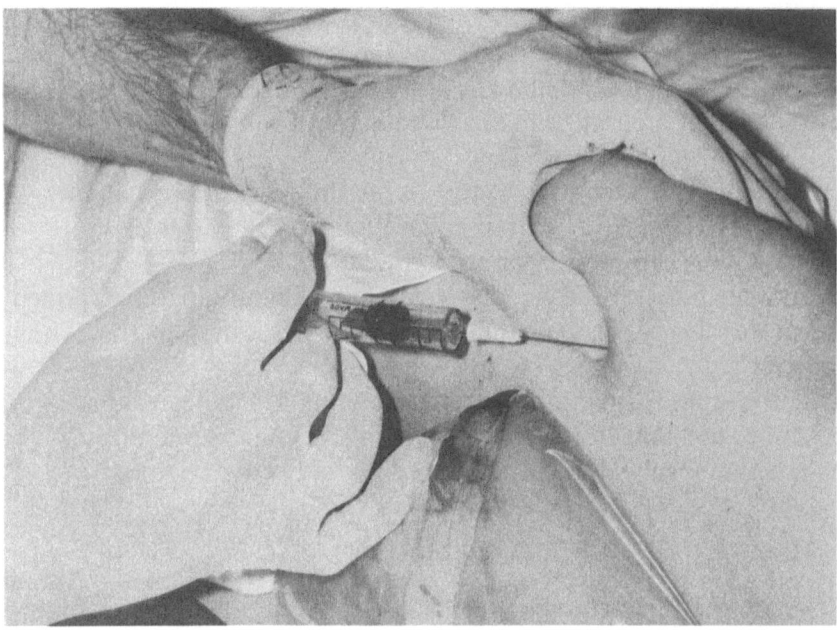

Fig. 4.2 The patella is held between the finger and thumb whilst being drawn laterally to increase the potential joint space for puncture. The skin is punctured over the patello-femoral groove beyond the tip of the thumb.

with the thumb, just above the mid-point of the patella. Local anaesthetic is infiltrated into the soft tissues in front of the tip of the thumb (Fig 4.2). It is unnecessary to inject local anaesthetic into the joint space. The local anaesthetic needle is left in position whilst the arthrogram needle is obtained (the puncture site can be difficult to identify). One needle is exchanged for the other. using the previous approach of displacing the patella laterally to widen the synovial space (Fig. 4.3) whilst passing the needle horizontally. Undue force must not be employed or the articular cartilage may be damaged. A sensation of 'give' is felt as the needle passes through the capsule and it may just impinge on the articular

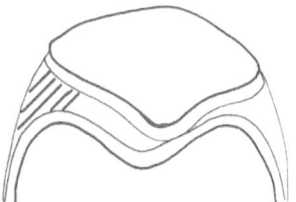
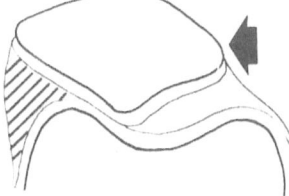

Fig. 4.3 Diagram to show the increase in size of the available joint space when the patella is directed laterally.

cartilage. Now it is necessary to establish whether the needle is in the joint space, although a large tense joint effusion will flow out spontaneously. The suprapatellar bursa is squeezed with the flat of the hand in order to identify smaller collections of fluid. If no fluid is present a check is made by injecting 10 ml air; it should inject easily.

Three ways of confirming that the needle is in the joint are available:

(a) during injection, the medial infrapatellar hollow will distend;

(b) after injection, air can be reaspirated freely;

(c) with the syringe, but not the needle, removed, the suprapatellar pouch is squeezed. Air will flow back through the needle if it lies freely in the synovial cavity.

The identification of some air within the joint on palpation indicates that air has entered at *some* time, not that the needle is *now* in the joint. Some air will often enter the joint spontaneously if it is punctured by a needle.

4.1.1 Comments

(i) The lateral side of the joint is no more difficult to puncture than the medial and it has the great advantage of proximity to the operator.

(ii) Many arthrographers do not use local anaesthesia. Its use has an advantage in training radiologists and, if it is desired to deflate the knee at the end of the examination, the area is still anaesthetized and the final needle puncture is painless. However, those who are invariably successful and do not apply the golden rule ('what would I like if I were the patient?') need not use local anaesthetic.

(iii) Some radiologists use smaller needles (21 gauge) for the joint puncture, which is entirely acceptable so long as an effusion is not present. Aspiration of fluid through a small needle is, however, a tedious exercise.

(iv) General anaesthesia is reserved for very small children (less than 4 years) and the occasional terror-stricken adult.

(v) Puncture employing local anaesthesia is virtually painless. Occasionally a patient will experience pain with the needle *in situ*, probably from contact with a synovial fringe. It is necessary to reposition the needle.

4.2 Injection of contrast medium

Any joint effusion is completely aspirated; persistence of fluid dilutes the medium and makes for an inferior examination. Maximal aspiration by gas displacement, as described by Ricklin *et al.* (1971), can be helpful, but is rarely necessary if the suprapatellar pouch is squeezed firmly. Next, 20 ml room air are injected and confirmation made that the needle is still in the joint cavity. The syringe is exchanged for one containing 3 ml Conray 280. After checking that the needle is still in the joint by aspirating air, the positive contrast medium is injected into the joint.

The syringe is removed and the connecting tubing attached to the side-arm of the stop-cock. The other end (now becoming unsterile) is passed to the assistant who connects it to the reservoir containing carbon dioxide. The 20 ml syringe is attached to the stop-cock and the stop-cock to the needle and a succession of boluses of 20 ml carbon dioxide are injected until the pressure within the joint slowly pushes out the plunger of the syringe. It is not possible to define a set amount of gas, it varies from patient to patient, depending on the size of the synovial space. If the patient has had a large effusion it could exceed 150 ml. An average volume would be 80 to 100 ml.

The needle, tap and syringe are removed in one movement by gripping the needle. An adhesive dressing is applied. The knee is flexed once – it should gurgle. If the knee was dry before puncture, this usually indicates that the contrast medium has been correctly injected into the joint space.

4.2.1 Comments

(i) Other studies have recommended the injection of varying amounts of positive contrast medium. Too little fails to coat the joint, too much pools and obscures the view. I have experimented with between 1 and 6 ml and find 3 ml generally satisfactory. The amount may be reduced in small children and increased in the presence of large synovial cavities.

(ii) Distending the joint with gas is essential. All other techniques, such as binding the suprapatellar space in the presence of a smaller volume of intra-articular gas, seem less satisfactory in achieving a good double-contrast result.

(iii) Carbon dioxide (together with the 20 ml air) (Butt and McIntyre, 1969) persists for about the right time. If air alone is used, it is politic to aspirate it on completing the procedure, as an uncomfortable amount will remain and some may still be present 10 to 14 days later. Oxygen produces similar slow absorption. As it is, with the air/CO_2 mixture, some patients can still feel the gas in their knees after 2 days, although disability from this cause is non-existent (Fig. 4.4).

(iv) Every once in a while, gas will lie in the joint, but the positive medium will be in the lateral periarticular tissue. It is assumed that the needle has become displaced or its bevel has passed incompletely into the joint. The extra-articular medium will not interfere with the examination; more contrast medium is injected into the joint. In some centres, contrast medium is always injected under fluoroscopic control.

(v) In dealing with children without joint effusions, it is sometimes best to perform the whole injection through the 25 gauge needle, as this is accepted more readily than a change to another, larger, needle.

(vi) In patellectomized patients it is also advisable to use the smaller needle. The quadriceps tendon is gripped between the fingers and thumb of one hand at the

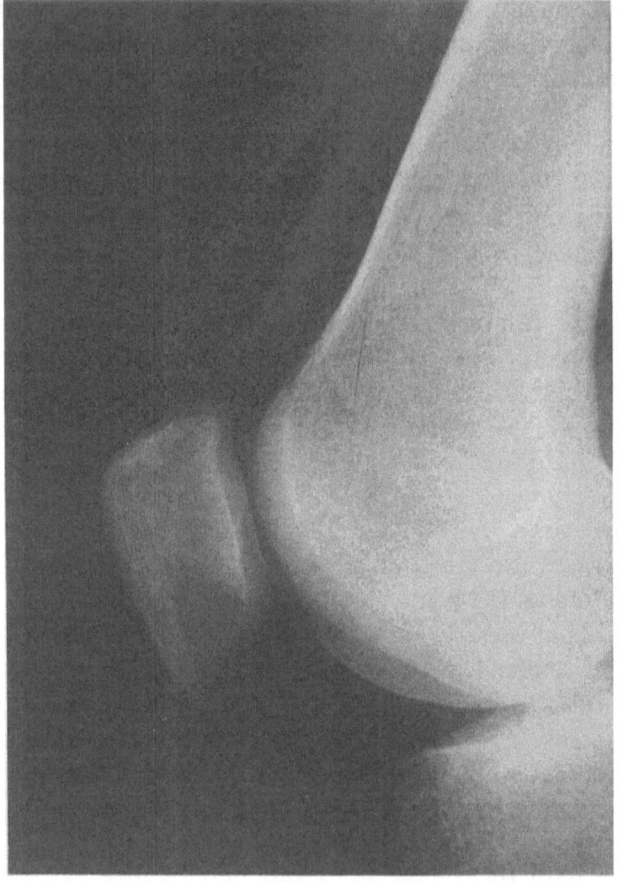

Fig. 4.4 Film showing as (remaining from an air/CO_2 mixture) in the suprapatellar pouch 5 days after a double-contrast arthrogram.

patellar level, whilst infiltrating with local anaesthetic. It is advisable to check that the needle is in the joint space on these occasions by injecting a small amount of positive contrast medium under fluoroscopic control. The medium will flow away from the needle and outline the tibio-femoral joint space.

(vii) Sometimes, although the needle is in the joint space, only a small amount of air is accepted. Reasons for this include:

(a) failure of the patient to relax; determined quadriceps contraction can prevent air entering the suprapatellar pouch;

(b) the suprapatellar pouch does not communicate with the joint (rare);

(c) the suprapatellar pouch is incompletely septate and a valvar mechanism is present. Flexion and extension of the knee may allow air to enter;

(d) the joint capacity is reduced ('frozen' knee) by pericapsulitis secondary to infection or trauma, including previous arthrotomy. If possible, the capacity is recorded and a search made for adhesive synovial bands during the arthrographic examination.

4.3 Preparation for fluoroscopy

The patient is next encouraged to stand on the floor; the knee will feel peculiar, but function normally. The patient should be under close surveillance at this stage as, occasionally, syncope occurs, as in all examinations involving skin puncture. It is recommended that a few steps are taken by the patient to encourage coating of the synovium by the medium. Vigorous exercise or 'pumping' the knee is unhelpful as it tends to produce bubbles which obscure the radiographic anatomy.

Whilst the patient has left the table this is prepared for fluoroscopic radiography. A box covered with a thin foam mattress (Fig. 4.5) is placed on the cephalic half

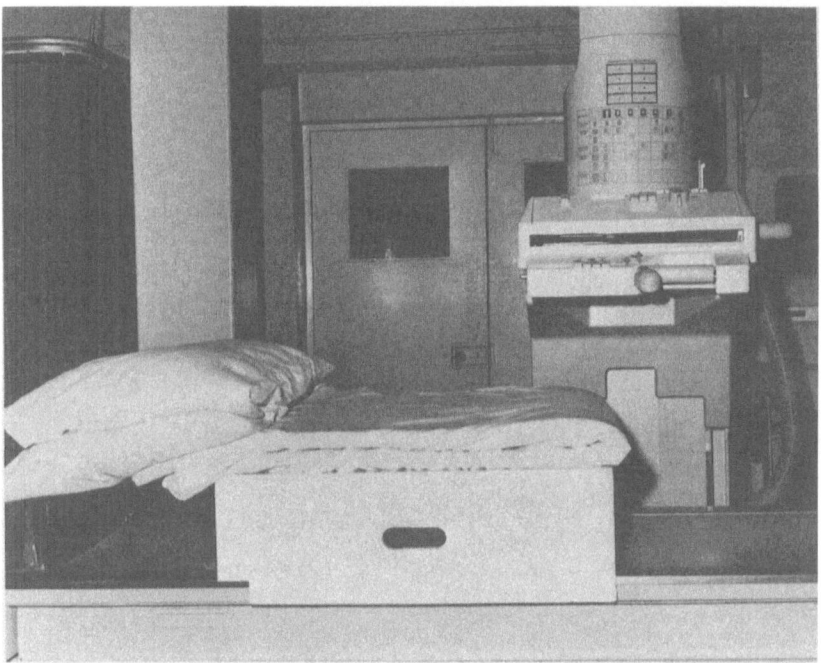

Fig. 4.5 Box for use in knee arthrography. The patients lies prone with his head on the pillow and his knee just beyond the edge of the foam mattress.

of the table. X-ray tables vary, so it is advisable to have one made to measure to ensure its stability. The height of the box should permit clearance of the patient by the fluoroscopic screen at its highest point. With most fluoroscopic apparatus this permits the use of a box 8 to 10 in. (20 to 25 cm) high. The construction should be sufficiently robust to support a large man.

The examination is performed with the patient prone, with the knee under examination just projecting over the edge of the box. It is recommended that a firm pad (about 10 cm deep) be placed under the distal thigh to keep the knee orthograde to the X-ray beam.

A canvas band (6 to 8 cm wide) with or without a metal loop, but with Velcro fixation, is used as a device for stressing the knee. Such a device is crucial to good arthrography. The one described here has the merit of effectiveness, variable size, simplicity and cheapness (Fig. 4.6). The band is looped round the patient's limb,

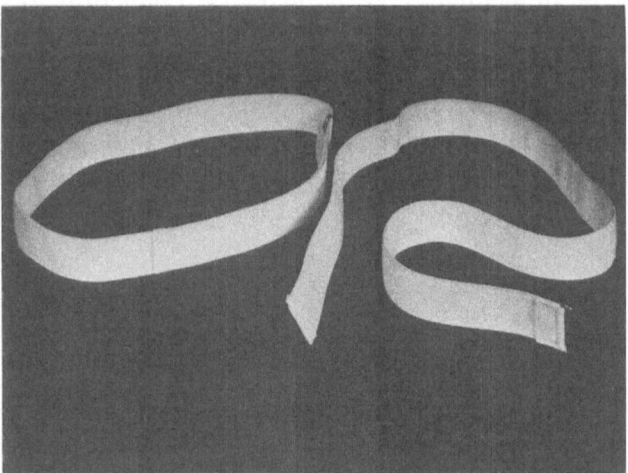

Fig. 4.6 Traction bands for use in knee arthrography. In this type, the end of the band passes through the metal ring and is then fastened by Velcro strips.

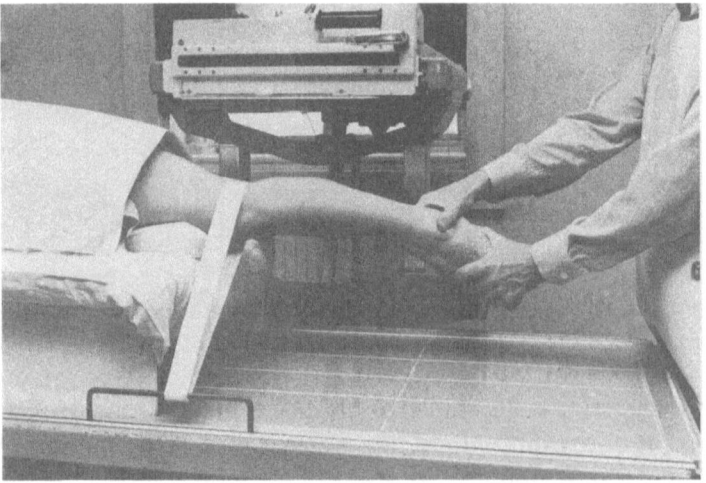

Fig. 4.7 *Position of the knee in arthrography*. The anterior horn of the left lateral meniscus is being examined. The knee is slightly flexed, the leg is externally rotated and varus stress is being applied.

just above the knee, passed through a metal slide or some other fixture at the edge of the table top and tightened. This band acts as a fulcrum, by means of which valgus or varus stress is applied to the knee, so that the tibio-femoral articular surfaces on the side to which the band is fixed separate as gas enters the side of the knee joint under examination (Fig. 4.7).

4.3.1 Comments

(i) Raising the patient above the level of the fluoroscopic table allows an increase in the focus–film distance and a consequent increase in the sharpness of the image. Use of a pillow alone is scarcely sufficient and does not even allow the patient's foot to clear the table.

(ii) Some arthrographers (Roebuck, 1977), a minority, perform the examination with the patient supine. One disadvantage of this position is that control of knee movements is less satisfactory. With the patient prone, the knee is extended unless the radiologist decides otherwise. In the supine position, flexion is difficult unless the patient is raised on a box, when the radiologist has to support the leg to maintain extension.

(iii) Stressing the knee is an integral part of the examination. Doing this manually (Ricklin *et al.*, 1971) is tiring and any inadvertent movement is difficult to control. Other mechanisms used for knee restraint include a metal flange (Angell, 1971) and slings with jam cleats (Levén, 1974).

4.4 Technique of radiological examination

4.4.1 The menisci

Earlier double-contrast techniques were purely radiographic (Nicholas *et al.*, 1970) and depended upon direction of the beam tangentially to the tibial condyle. Fluoroscopy provides a dynamic examination of the menisci, the movements of which are observed and spot films are obtained to record findings, sometimes in greater detail. This principle is similar to that employed in barium examination of the duodenal cap. Each meniscus is examined in turn, beginning with the medial meniscus unless a tear of the lateral meniscus is suspected. A routine fluoroscopic examination of the whole meniscus is obligatory and we routinely begin with the anterior horn. This means that the lower limb is fully internally rotated. For a child or young adult this movement can be achieved without difficulty by hip rotation alone without moving the trunk. For other patients, the trunk must be turned in order to view the extremities of each meniscus. Thus, in examining the medial meniscus of the left knee, the patient is required to turn on to his left hip (i.e. to his right) for the demonstration of the anterior horn and on to his right hip for the posterior horn. These movements soon become routine with practice, but the

Table 4.2 Technique for knee arthrography – patient prone

Part being examined		Patient rotated	Traction
Right medial meniscus	anterior horn	to his left (lies on right hip)	Band attached to left side of table Traction → right
or			
Left lateral meniscus	posterior horn	to his right (lies on left hip)	
Left medial meniscus	anterior horn	to his right (lies on left hip)	Band attached to right side of table Traction → left
or			
Right lateral meniscus	posterior horn	to his left (lies on right hip	

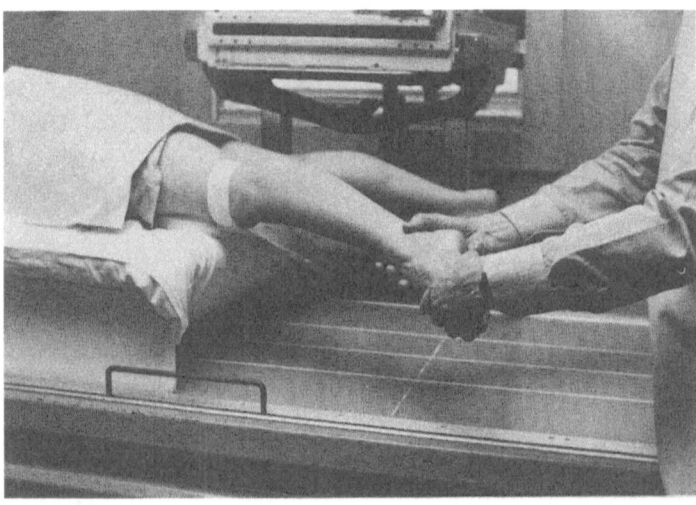

Fig. 4.8 *Position of the knee in arthrography.* Valgus stress being applied with the leg externally rotated to examine the posterior half of the medial meniscus of the left knee.

movements are given for the tyro in Table 4.2. Spot films are taken of each knee in eight positions during these manoeuvres. This means that although the whole of the meniscus is observed, its appearance is being recorded only in every 10 to 15° of rotation, as a total arc examined is probably not more than 110° because of overlap in front and behind, which obscures the extremity of each horn. Fortunately, this arc contains all the tears that are likely to have clinical significance. If any doubtful appearance is observed, further supplementary views are obtained.

In addition to rotation of the lower limb, the radiologist applies the appropriate varus or valgus stress (Fig. 4.8), so that gas enters the compartment so stressed, separating the meniscus from the condyles of the tibia and femur. The meniscus appears as a triangular wedge. Every attempt must be made to keep the image of the meniscus section in optimal profile ('orthograde' – Ricklin *et al.*, 1971). This can best be achieved by constant observation of the tibial plateau, which should also remain in profile (Fig. 4.9).

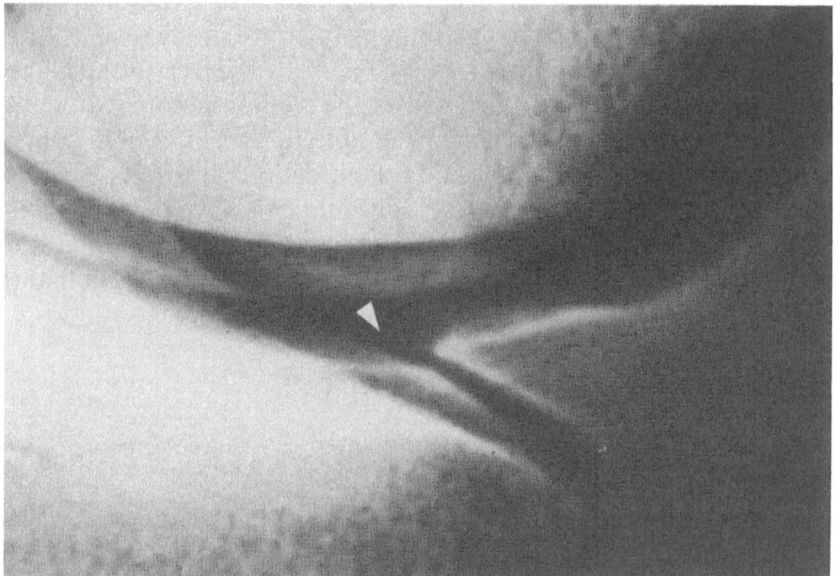

Fig. 4.9 *Anterior horn of normal medial meniscus.* The meniscus shows a triangular cross-section; both it and the tibial plateau are in profile. Note that the free edge of the meniscus can be visualized beyond the tip of the meniscal profile (arrow).

Examination of the medial meniscus is usually performed with the knee fully extended. The same sequence of positions and stress is performed to examine the lateral meniscus. The radiologist will find that slight flexion of the knee may be needed to obtain orthograde views of this meniscus in its anterior half.

4.4.1.2 Comments

Training radiologists in arthrography teaches that certain recurrent difficulties and problems arise. The radiologist should have a mental check list to apply when things are not satisfactory. Here are a few of the more common errors in technique.

(a) Wasting too much time on the anterior horn at the expense of the posterior horn. The anterior horn is easy to visualize. Perhaps two spot films of the anterior horn should be exposed, two of the middle third of the meniscus, leaving four views for the important posterior horn.

(b) Failure to examine the whole of the posterior horn, perhaps because of (a), to the point where the posterior condyles of the femur almost overlap. This sometimes results from insufficient rotation of the patient's trunk during the examination.

(c) Not stressing the knee sufficiently to achieve a double-contrast image. Such stress sometimes causes discomfort to the patient, but should not physically tax the operator. A firm steady pull is all that is needed, but check that the band has not slipped below the patient's knee. Anyone claiming that they are 'not strong enough' for a particular patient probably is using the leverage inefficiently. At the end of the examination, the spot films are inspected and any that are unsatisfactory are repeated until the examination is deemed to be comprehensive.

(d) Some authors claim either that it is not possible to obtain double-contrast films in all positions (Roebuck, 1977) or that loss of definition results if routine undercouch techniques are used. As a result, cassette tunnels have been employed (Peck and Butcher, 1974; Downes, 1979). The need for such complicated aids has never been apparent to me and the technique involves a retrograde step, in that the film is taken blind after fluoroscopy, rather than at fluoroscopy.

4.4.2 Ligaments and articular cartilage

4.4.2.1 Cruciate ligaments

The anterior cruciate ligament is examined routinely; the posterior cruciate ligament is formally examined only if damage is suspected. For the anterior cruciate ligament we have employed two methods.

(i) The patient sits with the thigh supported by a firm pad and the knee flexed to approximately 90°. Two films are taken with a horizontal beam technique (Fig. 4.10): one with the knee flexed and the second with the calf pressed into the edge of the table by active flexion of the knee.

(ii) With the patient lying on the side under investigation and using the fluoroscopic apparatus, films are obtained firstly at rest and secondly producing an anterior 'drawer' movement with a canvas band behind the upper calf pulling in the line of the anterior cruciate ligament, the knee being flexed to about 70°. During this procedure, the patient does not actively resist the movement, but relaxes the knee completely (Fig. 4.11).

We have no facilities for tomographic examination in the vertical plane (Mittler *et al.*, 1972), but can believe that this might improve the definition of the cruciate ligaments. Rupture of the anterior cruciate ligament may be difficult to diagnose clinically. Because they are extra-synovial, these ligaments can never be demonstrated in their entirety by arthrography. The leading edge of the anterior cruciate ligament, however, forms a sharp profile in the lateral projection and can be demonstrated regularly when it is normal. When it is torn, it occasionally can be

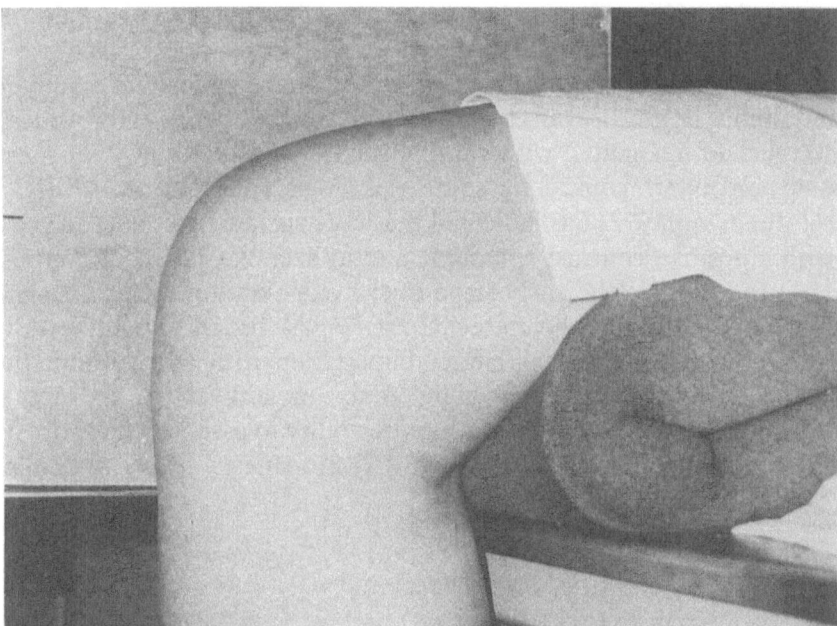

Fig. 4.10 Position of patient for evaluation of cruciate ligaments by horizontal beam technique. The patient is sitting on the X-ray table with the leg dependent.

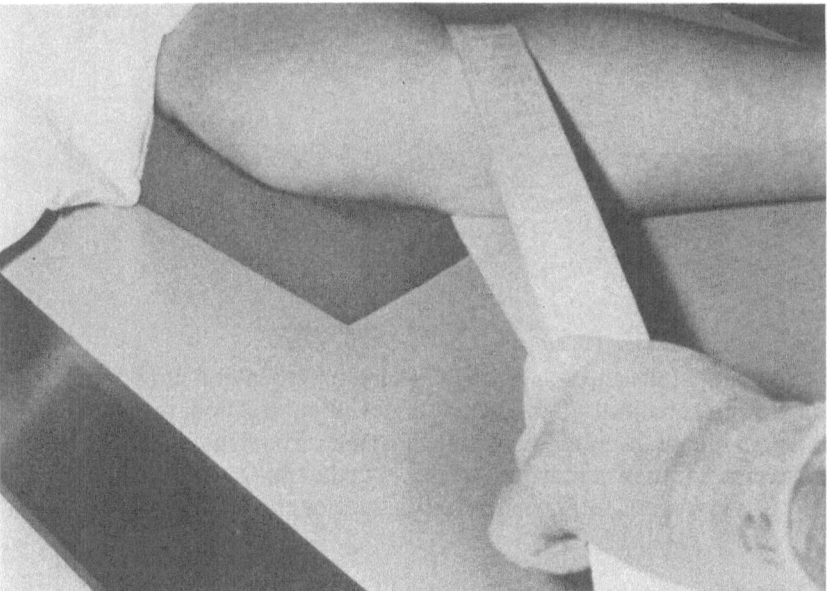

Fig. 4.11 The anterior drawer manoeuvre for demonstration of the anterior cruciate ligament. Traction on the band causes the tibia to move forward on the femur in the presence of ligamentous laxity. The radiologist's other hand (not shown) steadies the patient's leg by gripping the ankle.

observed as a worm-like filling defect, but more often its rupture is revealed at arthrography only by the failure to demostrate its margin.

Since arthrography was recommended as an aid to the diagnosis of ligament injuries by Lindblom (1938), a variety of methods have been employed to demonstrate the cruciate ligaments, with varying success. Frontal views show the ligaments crossing and are favoured by some radiologists (Roebuck, 1977).

Freiberger (Mittler *et al.*, 1972) has indicated that the cruciate ligaments are best demonstrated with a positive contrast technique and utilizes the excess of contrast medium pooling in the joint at the early stage of the examination. Such films are obtained by the use of a horizontal beam technique (Fig. 4.10). A dynamic study, which we have also favoured, employs lateral films taken with and without the application of the anterior drawer manoeuvre. This, in addition to the actual demonstration of the margin of the ligament, has the ability to assess its integrity by observing whether the ligament straightens with traction (Fig. 4.12). A similar

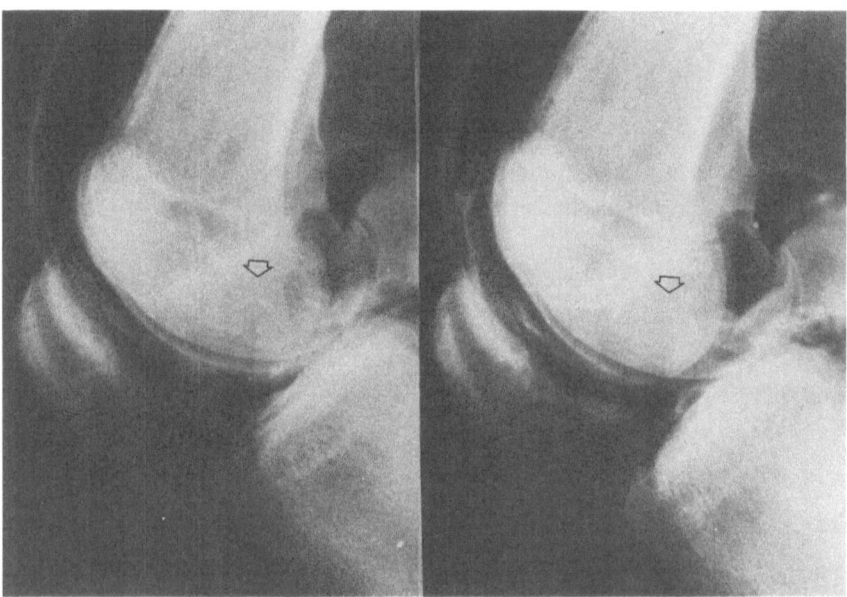

Fig. 4.12 Demonstration of the anterior cruciate ligament. Two lateral films of the knee during arthrography are illustrated. The left film, without traction, provides faint visualization of the margin of the anterior cruciate ligament. The right film has been obtained during an anterior drawer manoeuvre, in which the tibia and its cruciate attachment are drawn forward. The line of the intact anterior cruciate ligament is shown to straighten.

posterior drawer manoeuvre can be employed on the less frequent occasions when the posterior cruciate ligament's integrity is in doubt.

The difficulty of obtaining accuracy in the diagnosis of anterior cruciate rupture lies in the fact that the examination of the cruciates is, in most cases, an ancillary investigation secondary in importance to the demonstration of meniscal pathology.

When a primary single-contrast technique for cruciate delineation is used, arthrography can diagnose cruciate rupture in over 80 per cent of cases (Liljedahl *et al.*, 1965). In no series does the accuracy reach that obtained in tears of the menisci, for the anatomical reasons outlined earlier. It is also important to recognize that early diagnosis of such ligament ruptures is only of value to the patient where early surgical repair is practised.

Other techniques employed include tomography (Dalinka *et al.*, 1973; Firooznia *et al.*,1976) and xerography (Griffiths and D'Orsi, 1974). Even direct injection of the cruciate ligaments (Staple, 1972) has not proved successful.

4.4.2.2 Collateral ligaments
Tears of the capsule and the integral medial collateral ligament can, if so desired, be diagnosed in the acute stage by the demonstration of leakage of contrast medium into the peri-articular soft tissues. Such tears will naturally only be evident if the synovial lining is deficient and, as this has the ability to seal within a few days of injury, the absence of leakage of contrast does not exclude a capsular tear.

4.4.2.3 Articular cartilage and bursae
The articular cartilage can be observed covering the surfaces of the tibia and femur on the spot films. Its condition should always be recorded. Important features are thickness, surface regularity and absorption of contrast medium into the surface layers. In the diagnosis of chondromalacia patellae, quite striking claims have been made for arthrographic diagnosis. Horns (1977) in a series of 100 patients claimed an accuracy of 90 per cent in the diagnosis of lesions of the articular cartilage of the condyles and the patella. In a disorder which is ill understood and basically a clinical diagnosis, it would be wrong to suggest that such claims have general support. Indeed, in a careful arthrographic study of patellar chondropathy requiring a combination of lateral projections of the retropatellar region and three tangential views, Thijn (1976) found a correlation of his diagnosis of chondropathy in 74 per cent of cases, with an equal number (13 per cent) of false positive and false negative results. Much must depend on the technique used to determine reliability of the method. Arthroscopic diagnosis of chondromalacia is by no means infallible and many of such cases do not come to arthrotomy. As the name suggests, chondromalacia indicates softening of the articular cartilage and this, demonstrable only by direct pressure at arthrotomy, may be the only irrefutable early evidence. Absorption (imbibition) of contrast medium, when present, is certainly useful and suggestive evidence of damage to articular cartilage. We have, however, not found it a reliable or consistent sign.

The presence of a significant gastrocnemio-semimembranosus bursa should be recorded; sometimes the presence of a popliteal swelling is the patient's main complaint. If such bursae fill with positive contrast medium and obscure the medial meniscus, they can always be emptied by firm pressure with the patient prone whilst the knee is gently flexed and extended. In this position they will subsequently fill with gas. Apart from the common gastrocnemio-semimembranosus bursa, other bursae may be visualized from time to time. These are rarely very large and can be differentiated by their anatomical situation (Fig. 4.13).

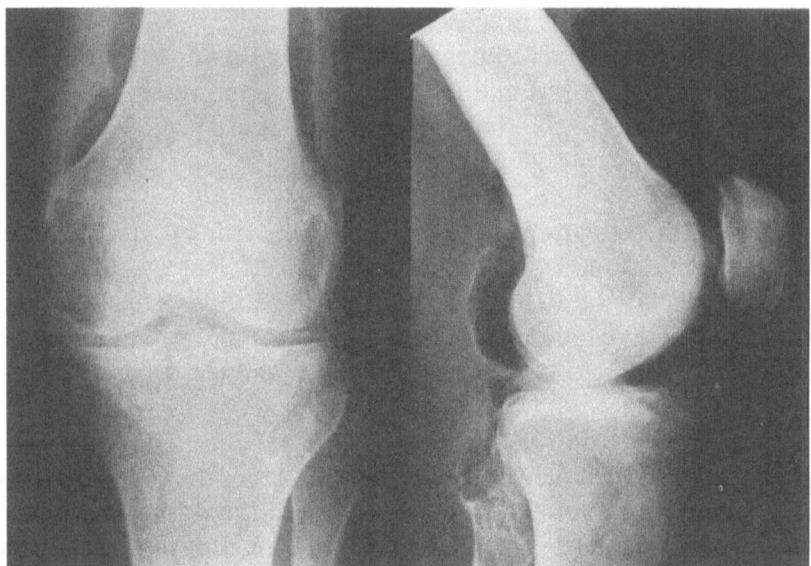

Fig. 4.13 Accessory bursa of the knee. Demonstration of this small normal sized bursa is an uncommon finding. It lies on the lateral side of the knee and is associated with the lateral head of the gastrocnemius.

4.5 Radiographic considerations

In the fluoroscopic arthrographic technique, the radiographer plays a major part, centring the part under examination and exposing the film whilst the radiologist positions the knee. For reasons of limiting the radiation dosage, the radiologist should retain control of the fluoroscopic foot-control, as only he knows when visualization is necessary. Communicating his wishes to a second party (the radiographer), who has the control switch, can double the exposure time.

The spot films not only record the appearances, but may reveal the presence or extent of a lesion not observed or correctly interpreted on fluoroscopy. They are, therefore, an integral part of the examination as well as a permanent record of the findings.

Some factors already mentioned will affect the radiographic quality, e.g. coating of meniscal and synovial surfaces, separation of the femoral and tibial condyles from the adjoining menisci and a prompt, decisive arthrographic technique. Other factors referred to already include the increase of the focus–film distance by elevating the patient on a box. Further technical considerations include:

(a) **focal spot.** This should be small. We prefer a 0.3 mm focal spot. An 0.6 mm focal spot is nearly as good and 1.0 mm can be perfectly acceptable, but the sharpness of objects is perceptibly reduced. When a focal spot larger than 1.0 mm is employed, the quality of the arthrogram becomes unacceptable.

Angell (1971) has detailed a means for conversion of standard fluoroscopic equipment, so that the smaller of the two focal spots provided can be employed for arthrography. These days, with improved equipment, most fluoroscopic machines are equipped with an 0.6 mm focal spot, or less, as a standard choice. As a consequence, the employment of a method using both under and over couch tubes should rarely prove necessary (Downes, 1979).

(b) **movement.** A blurred image due to movement by the patient is rarely a problem as generally the exposure time can be reduced to below 0.3s. In addition, firm positioning of the knee by the radiologist during the stress manoeuvre deters movement. Trouble only arises when the patient has a twitchy disposition and makes sudden unexpected movements.

(c) **grid.** Although it is probably possible to achieve adequate films whilst employing a grid, we dispense with it during arthrography. This naturally affects the discussion on film–screen combinations.

(d) **phototiming.** In my experience, automatic phototiming is unsatisfactory. The small field size in arthrography makes positioning so critical that it is impossible to achieve a consistent radiographic density.

(e) **collimation.** Correct collimation helps to reduce scatter and aids in the identification of abnormalities. Over-collimation results in loss of the required field of vision. An insert in the explorator with a suitable size of opening, e.g. 6 cm×4 cm, can act as a guide to correct collimation.

(f) **film–screen combinations.** Upon these depend the quality of the final product. Over the years we have changed our technique, our fluoroscopic machines, our focal spots, and with these, our films and screens. It is not, therefore, possible to lay down hard and fast rules or to predict what will be suitable in other radiological departments. It is, however, possible to state certain principles. The kilovoltage must be kept low, as in all soft tissue work, in order to maintain contrast. A moderately fast screen combined with a relatively high definition film is required. At the present time, we are employing mammographic films and screens (MR 50 – Agfa Gevaert). An exposure of an average size knee with this combination would be of the order of 44 kV, 200 mA and 0.24 s.

(g) **recording devices and markers.** No substitute for experience and practice exists in the orientation and reading of arthrogram films. Nevertheless, it would be churlish, now that our orthopaedic colleagues are at least interested in the technique, if we did not mark our films intelligibly. In most examinations, as a routine, four films are obtained, each comprising four exposures. Such films generally consist of the anterior medial, posterior medial, anterior lateral and posterior lateral segments. We use small inexpensive labels to identify each of these four films. A recently acquired fluoroscopic machine in our department exposes eight views on a 30 cm×24 cm film (Fig. 4.14). Unfortunately, the exposures do not

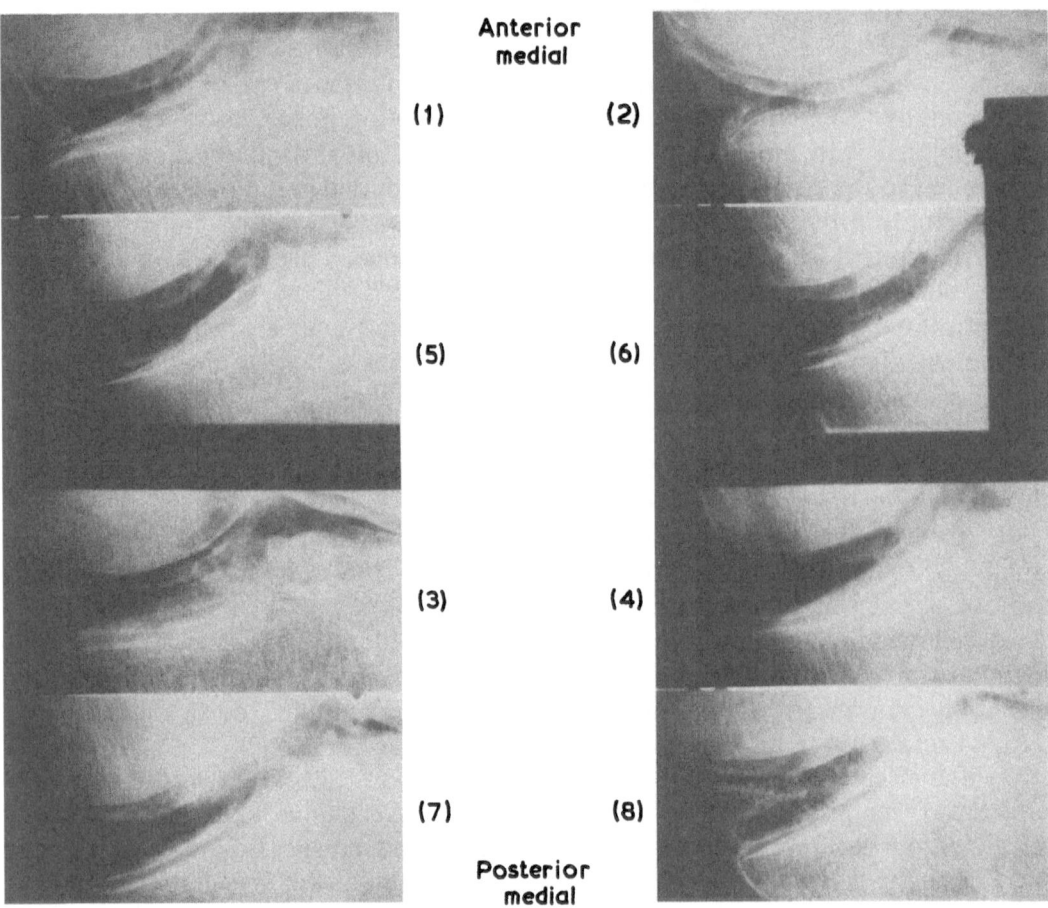

Anterior
medial

(1)   (2)

(5)   (6)

(3)   (4)

(7)   (8)

Posterior
medial

Fig. 4.14 Recording an arthrographic examination. Eight spot exposures have been recorded on a single 30 × 24 cm film. Such a facility can provide a significant reduction in the cost of film during arthrography.

follow a logical sequence, so we are obliged to number the spot films from in front backwards. By convention, the films are viewed as the menisci would be placed with the patient standing facing the radiologist.

A number of more sophisticated marking devices have been described (Russell and Lepage, 1976; Gerson and Griffiths, 1976).

References

Angell, F.L. (1971). Fluoroscopic technique of double contrast arthrography of the knee. *Radiologic Clinics of North America*, **9**, 85–98.

Butt, W.P. and McIntyre, J.L. (1969). Double-contrast arthrography of the knee. *Radiology*, **92**, 487–99.

Dalinka, M.K., Coren, G.S. and Wershba, M. (1973). Knee arthrography. *Critical Reviews in Clinical Radiology and Nuclear Medicine*, **4**, 1–59

Downs, M.O. (1979). New equipment for double contrast arthrography of the knee. *British Journal of Radiology*, **52**, 223–5.

Firooznia, H., Seliger, G., Baruch, H. and Weathers, R. (1976). Tomographic technique for visualization of the cruciate ligaments in double contrast arthrography. *Radiologic Technology*, **47**, 385–9.

Gerson, E.S. and Griffiths, H.J. (1976). A simple marking device for knee arthrography. *American Journal of Roentgenology*, **127**, 1057–8.

Griffiths, H.J. and D'Orsi, C.J. (1974). Use of xeroradiography in cruciate ligament injuries. *American Journal of Roentgenology*, **121**, 94–6.

Horns J.W. (1977). The diagnosis of chondromalacia by double-contrast arthrography of the knee. *J. Bone Joint Surg*, **59–A**, 119–120.

Levén, H. (1974). Arthrography of the knee with a modified technique. *Acta Radiologica Diagnosis, Stockholm*, **15**, 237–40.

Liljedahl, S.O., Lindvall, N. and Wetterfor, S.J. (1965). Early diagnosis and treatment of acute ruptures of the anterior cruciate ligament: a clinical and arthrographic study of 48 cases. *Journal of Bone and Joint Surgery*, **47–A**, 1503–13.

Lindblom, K. (1938). The arthrographic appearance of the ligaments of the knee joint. *Acta Radiologica*, **19**, 582–600.

Mittler, S., Freiberger, R.H. and Harrison-Stubbs, M. (1972). A method of improving cruciate ligament visualization in double contrast arthrography. *Radiology*, **102**, 441–2

Nicholas, J.A., Freiberger, R.H. and Killoran, P.J. (1970). Double-contrast arthrography of the knee. Its value in the management of 225 knee derangements. *Journal of Bone and Joint Surgery*, **52–A**, 203–20.

Peck, S.M. and Butcher, C. (1974). Apparatus for arthrography of the knee joint. *Radiography*, **40**, 46–7.

Ricklin, P., Rüttimann, A. and del Buono, M.S. (1971). *Meniscus Lesions*. Georg Thieme Verlag, Stuttgart.

Roebuck, E.J. (1977). Double contrast knee arthrography. Some new points of technique including the use of Dimer X. *Clinical Radiology*, **28**, 247–57.

Russell, E. and Lepage, J.R. (1976). Knee arthrography marker. *Radiology*, **118**, 460–2.

Staple, T.W. (1972). Extrameniscal lesions demonstrated by double-contrast arthrography of the knee. *Radiology*, **102**, 311–19.

Thijn, C.J. (1976). Double contrast arthrography in meniscal lesions and patellar chondropathy. *Radiologia Clinica (Basel)*, **45**, 345–62.

5 The normal arthrogram

A correct interpretation of the arthrographic appearances of the menisci implies that the radiologist is experienced in the technique and that not only is he able to identify normal appearances and a departure from them, but is also able to recognize a technically unacceptable arthrogram and to decline to make any deduction which is not supported by the appearances. Expertise in arthrographic interpretation cannot, therefore, be gained solely by reading books.

The menisci are not rigid structures, but soft and displaceable. It is for this reason that fluoroscopic examination has produced a great advance over static radiographs, which are now the record of the examination, not its *raison d'être*.

One complication that has been observed because of the plasticity of the menisci is deformation due to buckling, which must not be mistaken for meniscal damage (Hall, 1978).

The C-shaped configuration of the menisci makes it impossible to visualize their anterior or posterior extremities at arthrography. Both the posterior and anterior fat pads are projected over the menisci and at and beyond a true lateral position of the knee the contrast-outlined structures are superimposed. Fortunately, few tears are limited to these hidden regions of the menisci, as they are relatively protected from damage.

5.1 The normal medial meniscus

The medial meniscus is larger posteriorly than anteriorly and this is reflected in its cross-sectional area at arthrography. The meniscus shows a more or less triangular cross-sectional outline, of soft tissue density, with its pointed free margin directed towards the centre of the joint. It is deceptively easy to regard a meniscal view rather like a tomogram. It is, however, not a sectional picture and the free margin of the border of the meniscus is visible, stretching beyond the apex of the cross-sectional image (Fig. 5.1). The surface of the meniscus, coated with contrast medium, is smooth and initially the medium is not absorbed into the cartilage.

The cross-section of the anterior horn is an isosceles triangle (Fig. 5.2a), whilst

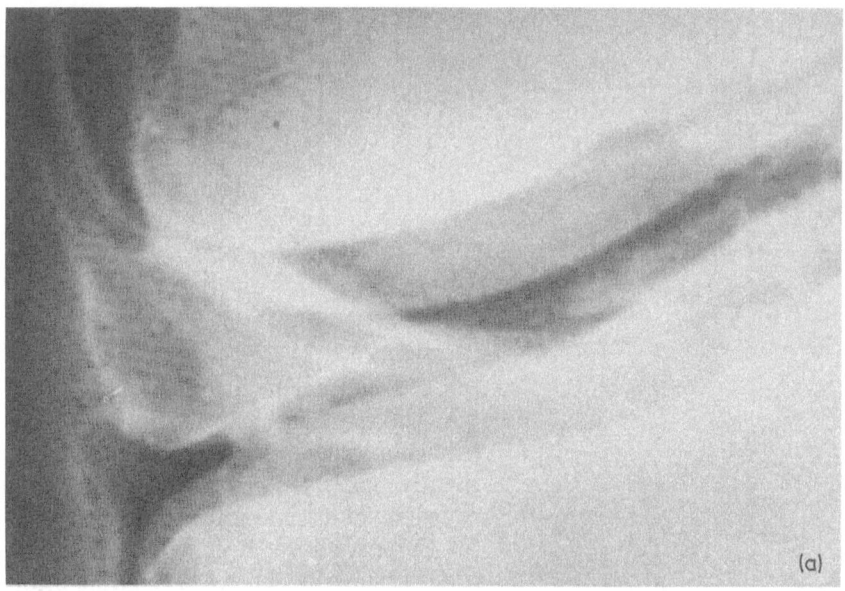

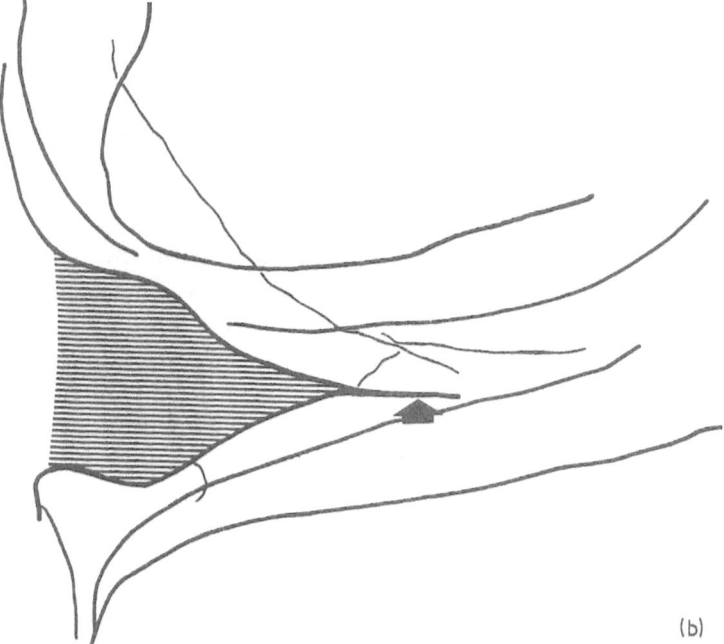

Fig. 5.1 *Normal anterior horn – medial meniscus*. The meniscal profile is shown (hatched area in (b)); the tibial plateau is also in profile. Other lines are formed by the meniscal border (arrow), the adjoining meniscal profile and synovial folds.

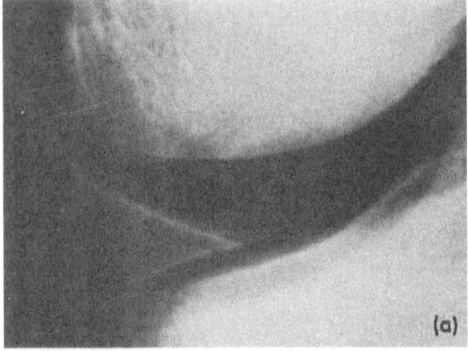
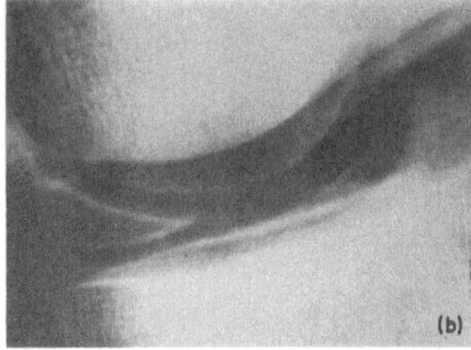
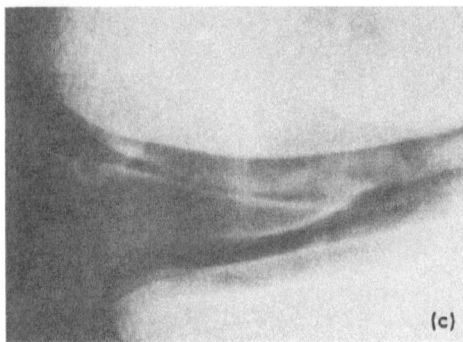

Fig. 5.2 Normal medial meniscus.
(a) Anterior horn, showing more or less triangular cross-section. (b) Middle third, slightly longer and flatter with a minimal concavity of its superior surface.
(c) Posterior horn, large, with a slightly concave superior surface, a small superior recess and a slightly convex inferior surface.

with the increase in size from in front backwards the posterior horn shows a slight concavity of its superior surface and a slight convexity of its inferior surface (Fig. 5.2c). No contrast medium should be observed within the meniscus or at its capsular insertion where its surface blends imperceptibly with the synovium. Peripheral recesses are observed at the margins above and below. These are usually small, but show considerable individual variation. Although when larger they are often wide and shallow, when they are deep and narrow thay may be indistinguishable from healed peripheral tears (Montgomery, 1974). The depth of a recess varies in any one patient and a prominent recess is never found along the whole length of a meniscus. These structures are developmental grooves related to the peripheral attachment of the menisci.

Menisci vary is size, shape and depth; a small or narrow meniscus is not necessarily abnormal if the other meniscus is similar in size. The same cannot be assumed when the surface is roughened or absorption of medium into the cartilage occurs, as this suggests an acquired traumatic lesion.

The synovial surface extends upwards to become continuous with the suprapatellar or paracondylar parts of the joint. Below, the synovial reflection is at the margin of the tibial articular surface. Frequently, the contrast-filled gastrocnemio-semimembranosus bursa overlies the posterior horn of the medial meniscus. It is rarely a problem unless filled only with positive contrast medium, when this must

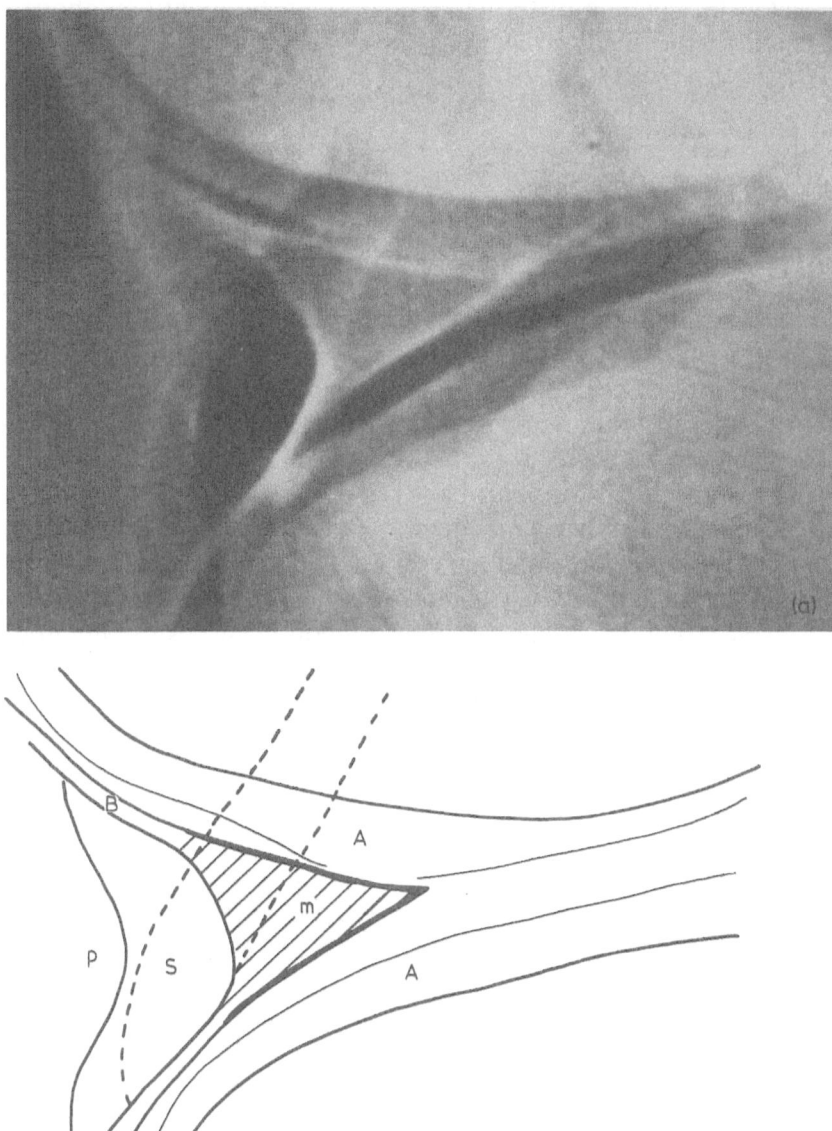

Fig. 5.3, (a) and (b) *Normal lateral meniscus – posterior horn.* Arthrographic appearance through the central part of the popliteus tendon sheath (S) showing the meniscus (m) attached by superior and inferior bands (B). Popliteus tendon (p) lies in the peripheral wall of the sheath; the continuation of the sheath is shown by the dotted lines passing obliquely upwards. Articular cartilage (A).

be displaced by gas. The opening of the bursa may often be identified above or within the substance of the medial meniscus.

5.2 The normal lateral meniscus

Unlike the medial meniscus, the size of the lateral meniscus changes little from front to back. Thus, the anterior horn is larger than that of the medial meniscus. The meniscus is more mobile than the medial meniscus. Its position in the joint space is influenced less by application of varus stress because of its looser peripheral attachments and their separation from the collateral ligament. For this reason it is often necessary to employ flexion of the knee to demonstrate that part of the meniscus between the anterior horn and the appearance of the anterior end of the popliteus tendon sheath. This latter structure is the hallmark of the lateral meniscus and must not be misinterpreted. Its features are: (a) a typical location in the posterior horn; (b) a smooth surface with bands above and below attaching the meniscus to the capsule. As has been mentioned earlier, a normal defect in the superior band is present anteriorly and in the inferior band posteriorly. The explanation for this is shown in Fig. 2.7. The cross-section of the tendon sheath can be round, oval or even rhomboidal. The popliteus tendon itself lies usually in the lateral wall of the sheath, into which it may bulge (Fig. 5.3). Extremely rarely, it may form a filling defect within the tendon sheath. The superior reflection of the synovium is the same on the lateral side of the joint as on the medial side. Inferiorly, in most subjects, the synovium is reflected onto the tibia several millimetres more distally than on the medial side (Fig. 5.4).

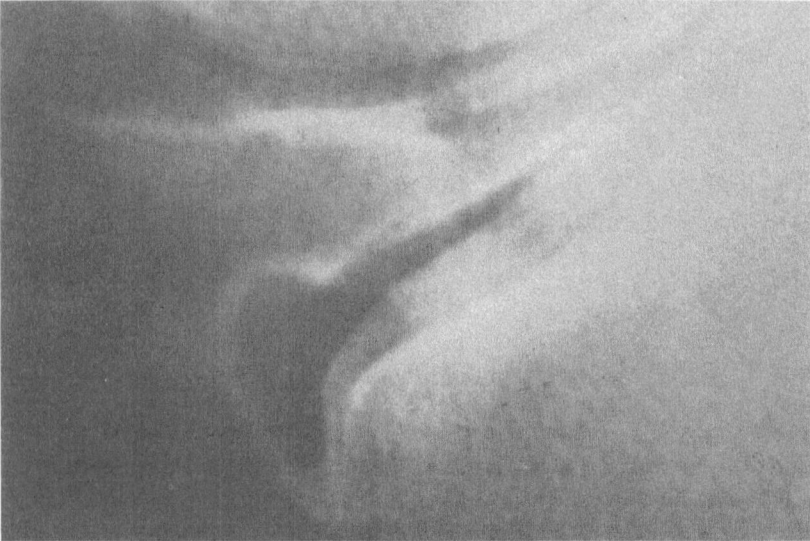

Fig. 5.4 Lateral meniscus to show the synovial reflection on the tibia anterior to the popliteus tendon sheath.

It is rare for any bursa on the lateral side of the knee to interfere with the demonstration of the meniscus. The popliteus bursa (the blind posterior end of the popliteus tendon sheath) is interposed between the posterior border of the tibia and the popliteus muscle and therefore tends to lie below the level of the meniscus.

5.2.1 *The normal joint space and articular cartilage*

The potential joint space of the knee becomes a true space during arthrography when it is filled with gas. Any structure, apart from the menisci, observed between the articular surfaces of the femoral and tibial condyles is abnormal and must be explained.

It is not possible to demonstrate all the articular cartilage of the femoral condyles during arthrography and, because of the concavity of the tibial plateau, even less of the tibial surface can be visualized. Nevertheless, articular cartilage is evident on each spot film and should be of uniform thickness, with a smooth surface and without localized absorption of contrast medium into its surface (Figs. 5.1 and 5.3).

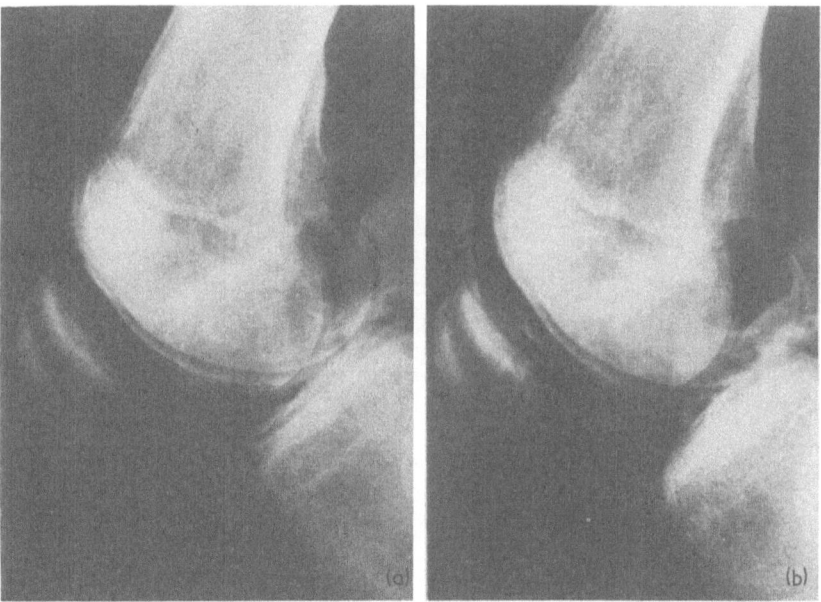

Fig. 5.5 Lateral arthrographic view showing (a) faint image of anterior cruciate ligament at rest. (b) During the anterior drawer manoeuvre, the margin of the anterior cruciate ligament becomes straight, indicating it is intact. The margin of the posterior cruciate ligament is visible, forming a tent-like appearance with the anterior ligament.

5.3 The normal cruciate ligaments

The radiological diagnosis of a completely normal anterior cruciate ligament can be made sometimes with absolute certainty. The ligament appears as a faintly curved line passing from the anterior part of the intercondylar area of the tibia upwards and backwards into the femoral intercondylar notch. With anterior traction on the tibia it straightens like a bowstring (Fig. 5.5). Although visualization of this is a common finding, only too often definition is poor for a variety of reasons; sometimes marginal evidence of laxity leads to indecision. For this reason, like others (Butt and McIntyre, 1969; Kaye and Freiberger, 1975), we have found it

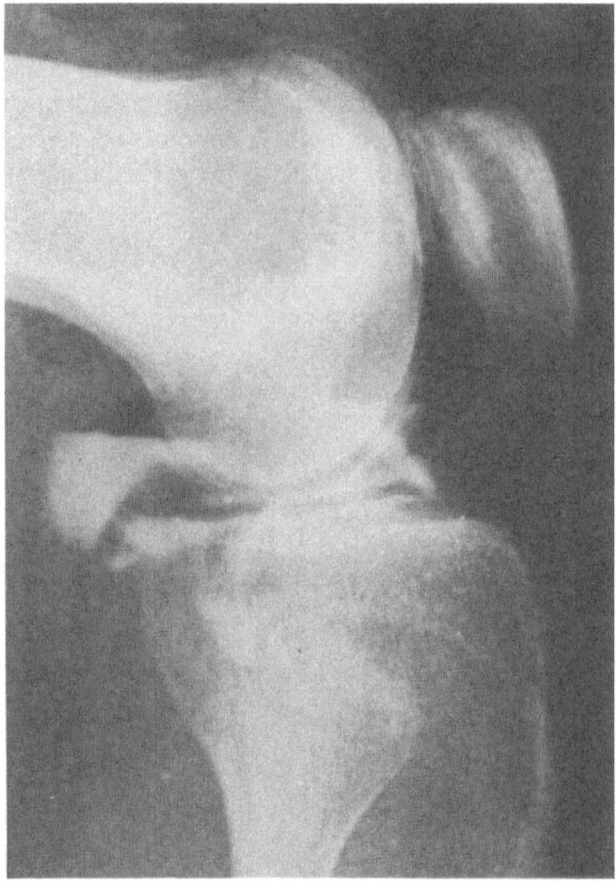

Fig. 5.6 *Anterior cruciate ligament.* The ligament is here demonstrated by the use of a horizontal beam technique, so that the pooling of positive contrast medium in the floor of the knee joint produces what is essentially a single-contrast examination in respect of the ligament.

difficult to achieve the accuracy of diagnosis in respect of the cruciate ligaments found in the assessment of the menisci. The use of a horizontal beam lateral film has been advocated as producing a greater accuracy in demonstration of the intact ligament (Mittler *et al.*, 1972) (Fig. 5.6).

Although, therefore, the absence of a shadow of the anterior cruciate ligament does not always indicate rupture, it is unusual for a ruptured ligament to show an entirely normal arthrographic appearance. This can only happen when the synovial covering of the ligament (which essentially produces the shadow) remains intact, whilst the ligament beneath is ruptured.

An infrapatellar synovial fold is normally found in the lateral arthrographic projection (Ricklin *et al.*, 1971). Dalinka and Garofola (1976) have drawn attention to the fact that this fold may simulate the anterior cruciate ligament, especially when the cruciate ligament is ruptured and the fold becomes more obvious.

Differentiation of the two structures is made by observing that the fold extends further forwards than the tibial attachment of the anterior cruciate ligament (Fig. 5.7)

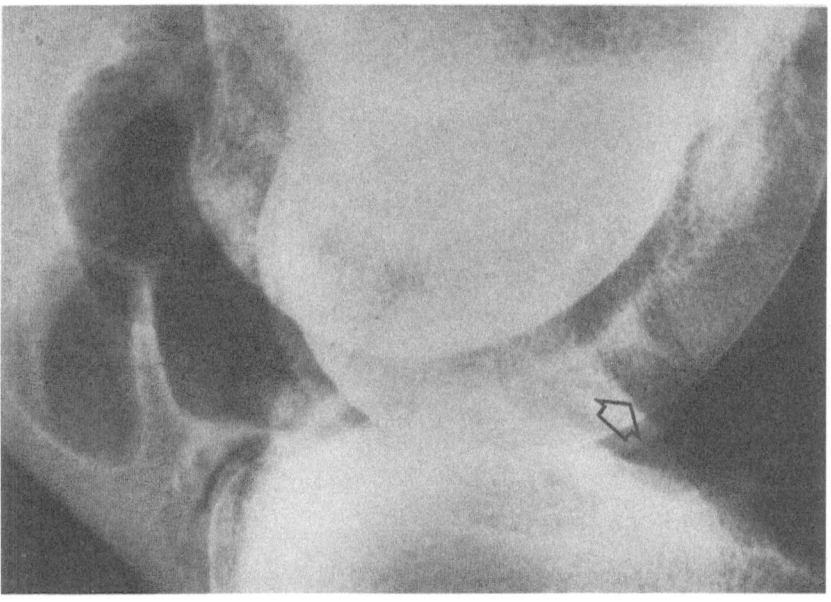

Fig. 5.7 Lateral view of the knee to show synovial fold (arrow) mimicking the anterior cruciate ligament, but reaching more anteriorly on the tibial plateau.

The posterior cruciate ligament arises from the posterior margin of the tibial intercondylar area. Its posterior synovial covering is frequently demonstrated, on the lateral arthrographic film, to form an oblique line which meets that of the anterior cruciate ligament in a tent-like manner (Fig. 5.5). Although a tear of the posterior cruciate ligament is rarely suspected or thought to be clinically important, Trickey (1968) believes it is a more common injury than is realized and especially prevalent in motor cyclists. If, as is indicated by reports in the literature (Trickey, 1968; Smillie, 1970), early operation is the treatment of choice, arthrographic demonstration of the ligament should be sought in injuries involving backward displacement of the tibia. In three-quarters of Trickey's cases, however, a fragment of bone was avulsed from the ligament's tibial attachment and this could be identified on the plain film (Fig. 5.8).

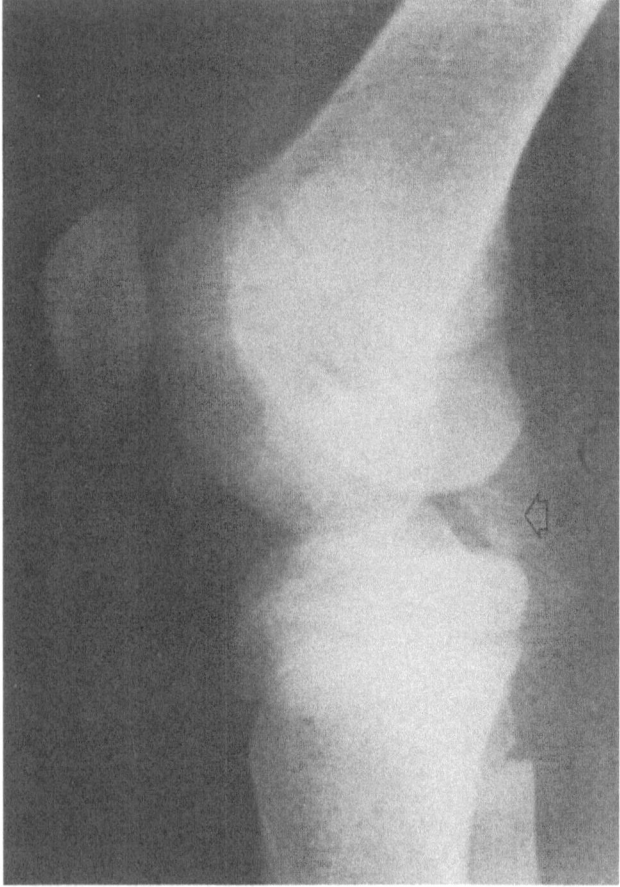

Fig. 5.8 *Avulsion injury of the posterior cruciate ligament.* A fragment of bone (arrow) is visible in the posterior compartment of the knee. It proved to be the tibial attachment of the posterior cruciate ligament. The patient was treated by surgical reattachment of the fragment, hence restoring the integrity of the ligament.

References

Butt, W.P. and McIntyre, J.L. (1969). Double-contrast arthrography of the knee. *Radiology*, **92**, 487–99.

Dalinka, M.K. and Garofola, J. (1976). The infrapatellar synovial fold: a cause for confusion in the evaluation of the anterior cruciate ligament. *American Journal of Roentgenology*, **127**, 589–91.

Hall, F.M. (1978). Buckled meniscus. *Radiology*, **126**, 89–90.

Mittler, S., Freiberger, R.H. and Harrison-Stubbs, M. (1972). A method of improving cruciate ligament visualization in double-contrast arthrography. *Radiology*, **102**, 441–2.

Kaye, J.J. and Freiberger, R.H. (1975). Arthrography of the knee. *Clinical Orthopedics*, **107**, 73–80.

Montgomery, C.E. (1974). Synovial recesses in knee arthrography. *American Journal of Roentgenology*, **121**, 86–8.

Ricklin, P., Ruttimann, A. and Del Buono, M.S. (1971). *Meniscus Lesions*. Georg Thieme Verlag, Stuttgart.

Smillie, I.S. (1970). *Injuries of the Knee Joint*, 4th Edn. Livingstone, Edinburgh.

Trickey, E.L. (1968). Rupture of the posterior cruciate ligament of the knee. *Journal of Bone and Joint Surgery*, **50–B**, 334–41.

6 Interpretation – the abnormal arthrogram

It is easy to say that, having established the normal appearances, everything else must be abnormal. The identification of normal appearances and their variations is perhaps the most difficult task in radiology, if not in medicine as a whole. To perform an arthrogram with reasonable dexterity takes a short time, to interpret the findings with competence and accuracy requires considerable experience with many arthrograms.

In his interpretation of an arthrogram, the radiologist is correlating the two-dimensional image with his knowledge of the three-dimensional anatomy. As each spot film is obtained in a slightly different position, it is possible for any lesion observed to be defined in both site and extent.

6.1 Tears of the substance of the meniscus

Although it is customary to classify tears into certain basic types, many, if not most, meniscal tears are complex. The arthrographer is even more aware of this fact than the surgeon, who does not see the whole meniscus *in situ* and cannot determine the course of closed tears deep in the meniscus by observing its external surface. It is, therefore, only possible to agree in part with some authors (Nicholas *et al.*, 1970; Dalinka *et al.*, 1973) that the type of tear cannot be accurately described by the arthrographic findings. Arthrography is practised in an orthopaedic surgical environment and if the surgeons consider that such tears can be described and classified at operation, it is essential to try and talk their language, remembering that the radiographic description can be the more accurate one.

All tears may show irregular rather than clean cleavage planes with oblique V or star-shaped cross-sections.

Radiologically, the following classification can be employed (Fig. 6.1).

(1) **Vertical tears (a)**
    (i) Simple short closed tears which may be partial or complete.
    (ii) Long vertical tears which, when they extend forward to allow displacement of the central fragment, constitute 'bucket-handle' tears.

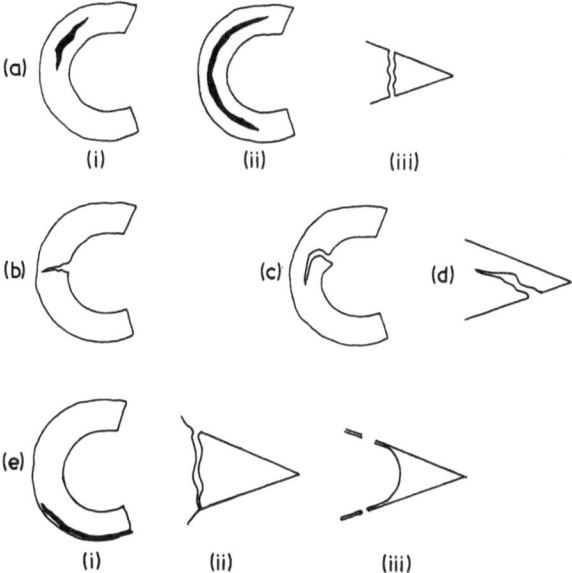

Fig. 6.1 *Diagram of types of meniscal tears*. (a) Vertical tears: (i) limited tear; (ii) long bucket-handle tear; (iii) profile view of vertical tear. (b) Radial tear. (c) Parrot-beak tear. (d) Profile of horizontal cleavage tear which has reached the undersurface of the meniscus. (e) (i) and (ii) Peripheral tear (detachment) of medial meniscus. (iii) Peripheral detachment of posterior horn of lateral meniscus. Profile view to demonstrate deficient bands.

(2) Radial tears (b).

(3) Parrot-beak and other complex tears. In these, a combination of vertical and radial elements results in detachment of one end of the tear with possible displacement. It is clearly impossible to determine whether the tear depicted in Fig. 6.1 (c) began vertically or radially. Experience may suggest the likely manner in which this lesion arose as a result of multiple traumatic incidents, but this is conjecture.

(4) Horizontal tears ('degenerative cleavage tears') (d).

(5) Peripheral detachment. These frequently involve the posterior horn. On the medial side the tear takes place through the outermost part of the meniscus or the menisco-capsular junction (e (i) and (ii)), whilst on the lateral side detachment occurs as a result of rupture of the bands on either side of the popliteus tendon sheath (iii).

The radiologist is able to define the extent of the tear by observing whether it involves the anterior, middle or posterior thirds of the meniscus. When the tear is confined to the anterior or posterior horn this should be stated.

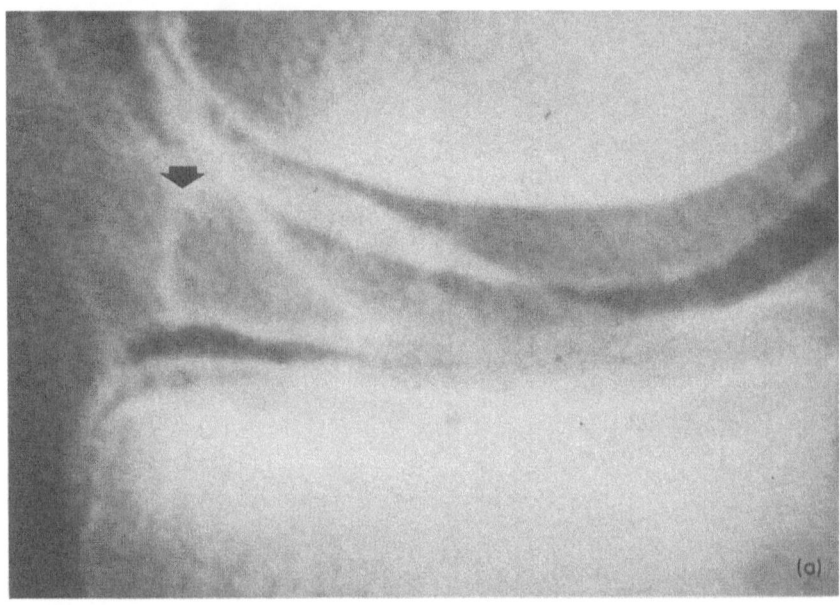

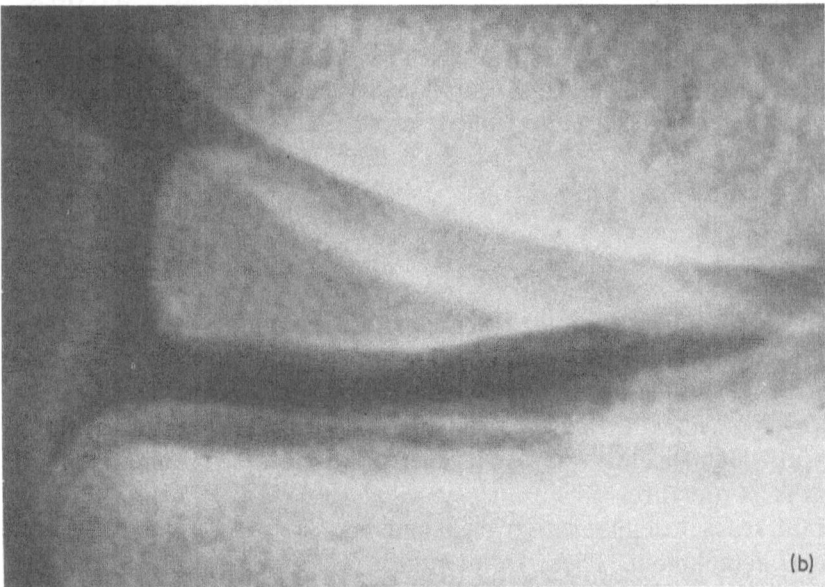

Fig. 6.2 (a) and (a) *Bucket-handle tear of medial meniscus*. A 17-year-old female water skier was examined following a hyperextension injury to her left knee. A tear of the medial meniscus was suspected. The arthrogram shows a widely separated vertical tear of the posterior horn (a), which extends into the anterior horn as a closed tear (b) (arrow).

6.1.1 Vertical (longitudinal) tears (Fig. 6.1, a)

These are the commonest form of meniscal injury in the young adult. The medial meniscus is damaged more often than the lateral and a vertical tear of its posterior horn is the common meniscal lesion. A tear is defined by the presence of contrast medium within the substance of the meniscus. A closed tear may accept only a thin film of positive contrast medium. The radiologist should, by the appropriate stress manoeuvre, open the tear and cause gas to pass into the cleft in addition, as this provides confirmation that a tear exists.

Wide separation at the site of the tear indicates either that the tear is a long one ('bucket handle') (Fig. 6.1, a (ii)) or that one end of the tear has broken through the free margin (Fig. 6.1, c). It must be emphasized that it is not always possible to distinguish with certainty whether a bucket-handle tear is closed or open, although change in direction, widening (Fig. 6.2) or blurring of the outline at the extremity of a tear may suggest a free flap of meniscus.

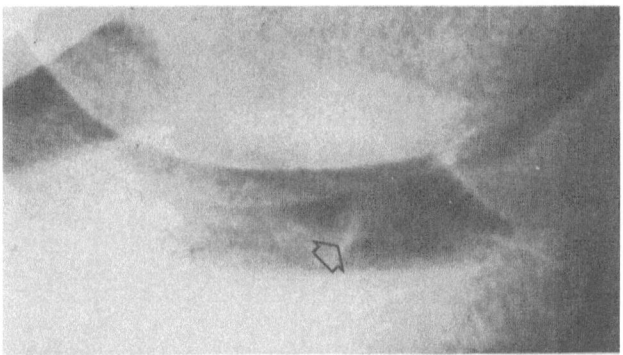

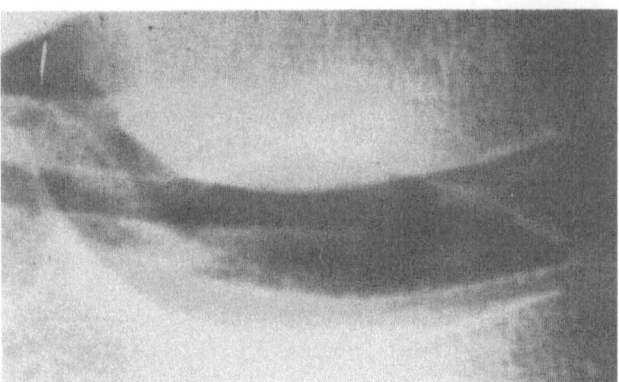

Fig. 6.3 *Tear of medial meniscus*. The cross-sectional area of the meniscus is abnormally small. In this case, the detached meniscal fragment is visible on the surface of the tibial plateau (arrow).

Reduction in size of the meniscal cross-sectional area is not necessarily abnormal, but any associated change in the normal triangular shape of the meniscus suggests damage, particularly if it is localized. Such an appearance may indicate the complete detachment of a segment of free meniscal edge (Fig. 6.3). Failure to demonstrate the fragment is not unusual; it may have resorbed completely (Ricklin *et al.*, 1971) or may have passed into the 'silent' intercondylar area, where it can

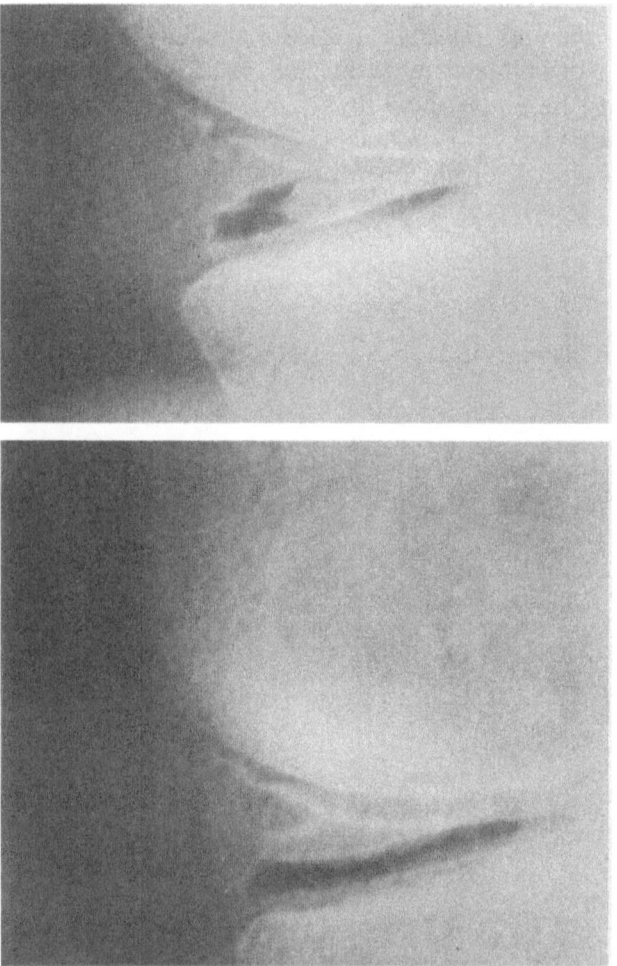

Fig. 6.4 *Tear of posterior horn of medial meniscus.* Although classified for convenience as vertical, this tear is oblique. In the lower film it is closed, whilst in the upper one separation has occurred, suggesting that the tear may have produced a complete detachment at its posterior extremity.

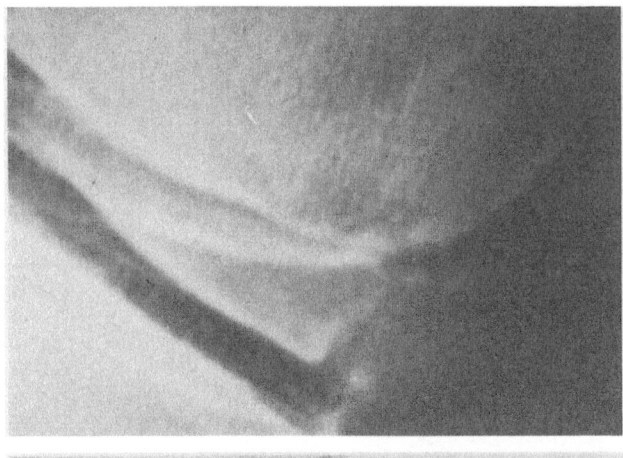

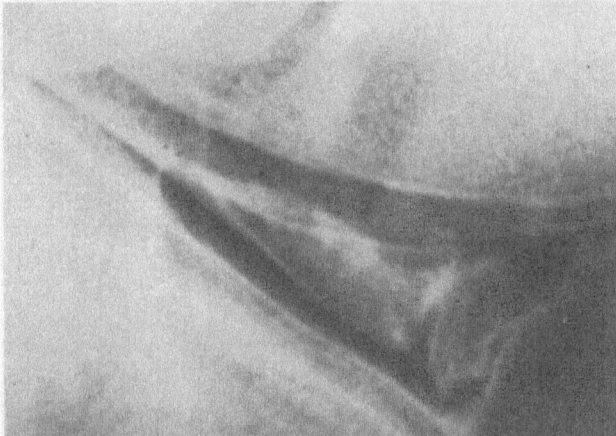

Fig. 6.5 *Tear of posterior horn of medial meniscus.* A
vertical tear is shown in the upper film. In the lower
film, from a more posterior situation, the tear has a
double vertical configuration. The possibility of leaving
a fragment behind at operation has to be taken into
account and the surgeon advised of the specific nature
of the tear.

become adherent to the synovial lining and cause no symptoms. Examples of
vertical tears are shown in Figs. 6.4 to 6.7.

6.1.2 Radial tears (Fig. 6.1, b)

These are difficult to demonstrate arthrographically because the tear lies
perpendicular to the X-ray beam. The meniscus on either side of the tear appears
normal at arthrography. The radiologist should suspect such a lesion when the

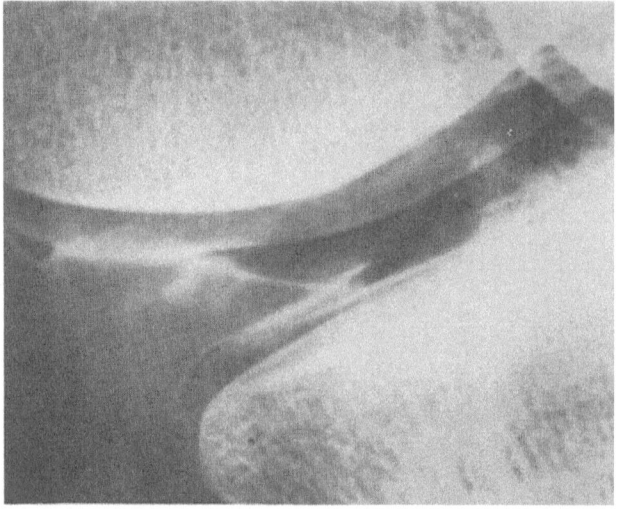

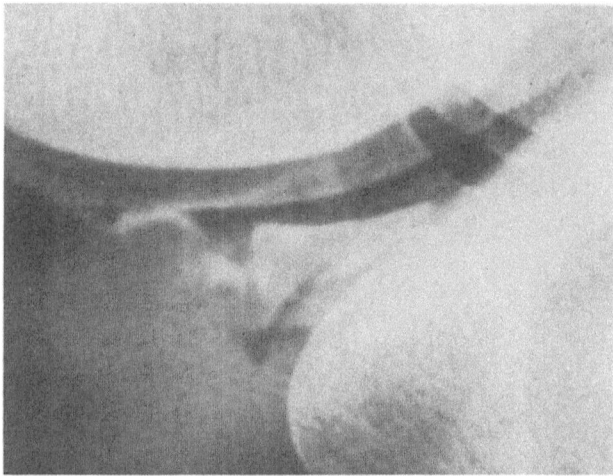

Fig. 6.6 *Peripheral vertical tear of posterior horn of medial meniscus.* Both films are of the posterior horn (note the superimposition of the femoral condyles). The tear is, however, only clearly delineated on the lower film. The importance of always visualizing the whole of the posterior horn of the meniscus cannot be overemphasized.

meniscus inexplicably fails to respond to an adequate stress manoeuvre, remaining adherent to the condylar surfaces due to loss of tension in its long axis occasioned by the tear (Fig. 6.8). Fortunately, a simple radial tear is most uncommon; it is commonly combined with a short vertical tear to form a flap ('parrot beak' tear) (Fig. 6.1,c) and this vertical element is easier to identify.

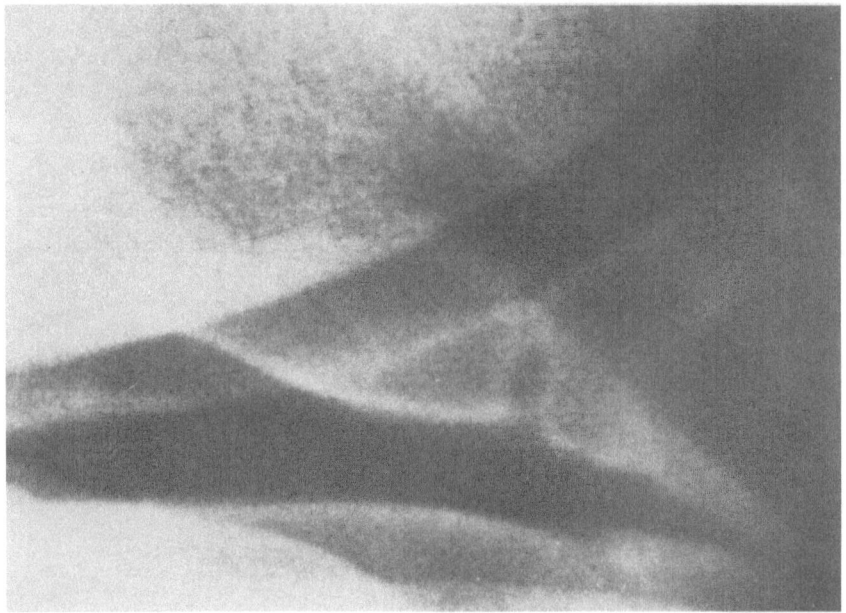

Fig. 6.7 *Vertical tear of the posterior horn of the lateral meniscus.* The tear is visualized as completely distinct from the popliteus tendon sheath and is comparable to the vertical tear of the posterior horn of the medial meniscus, although very much less common.

This type of tear is most commonly found in the middle third of the lateral meniscus and has been considered to be the result of central cystic degenerative change within the meniscus (Smillie, 1970). This variety of tear should also be suspected when a 'step' or discrepancy in size is observed between the central and peripheral portions of the meniscus at arthrography (Fig. 6.9 a, b).

6.1.3 Complex tears

These are common and are formed by a combination of vertical, radial and/or horizontal tears.

Detached fragments or generalized fragmentation of the meniscus may be seen and no conclusion as to the mechanism involved can be made. In such cases, the arthrogram often underestimates the size of the tear observed in the surgical specimen (Fig. 6.8).

6.1.4 Horizontal tears

The generally accepted pathology of horizontal (cleavage) tears is one of degenerative change in the fibrocartilage of the meniscus. Loss of elasticity and

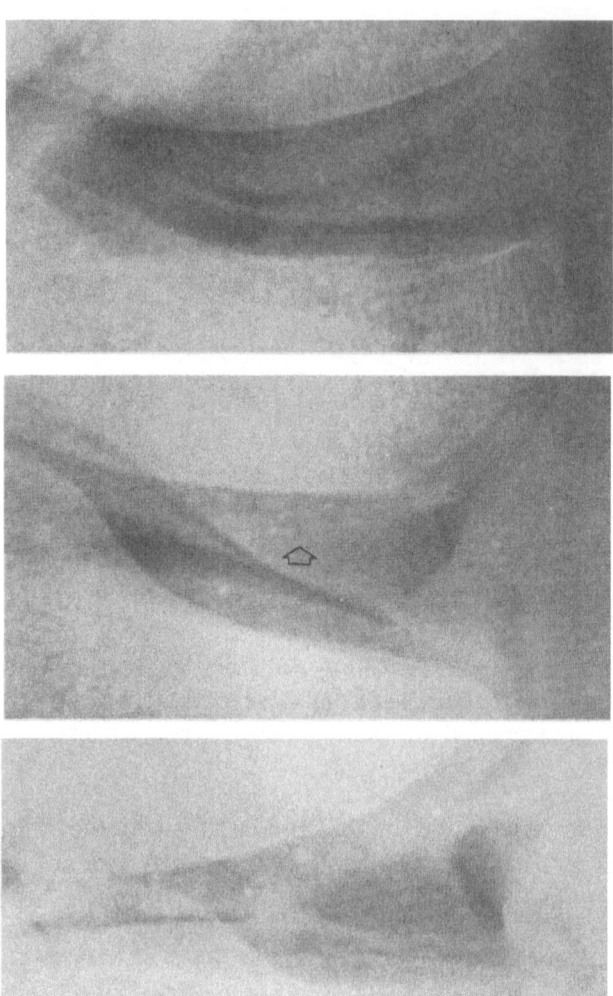

Fig. 6.8 *Tear of lateral meniscus.* This 25-year-old man sustained a twisting injury to his knee at football and a tear of the lateral meniscus was suspected. At arthrography, considerable difficulty in demonstrating the lateral meniscus was experienced (in itself a suspicious observation). Although the meniscus tended to adhere to the femoral condyle, a tear of its superior surface was observed (arrow) and reported. At operation, a parrot-beak tear of the middle third of the meniscus was found.

mobility causes movement to take place, not between the femur and superior surface of the meniscus, but between the meniscus and the tibial condyle,

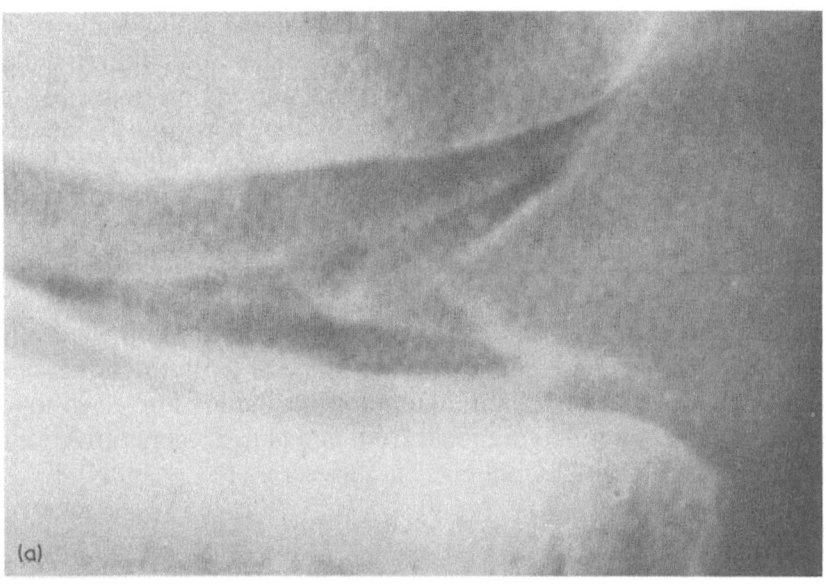

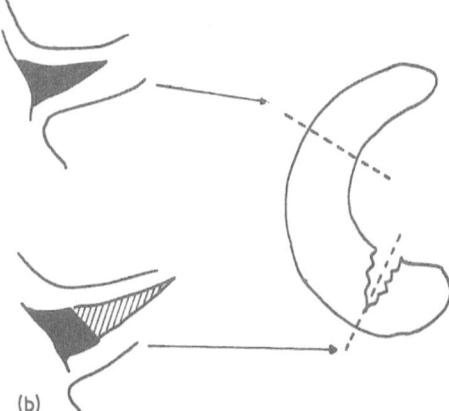

Fig. 6.9 *Complex ('parrot-beak') tear.* (a) The combination of a vertical and radial direction in such a tear may result in difficulty in the definition of the injury. Here, an oblique tear is shown but, in addition, the detached free edge is poorly visualized as a consequence of the radial element. (b) The diagram illustrates how the arthrographic appearances can produce a step at the margin of the radial tear and reduced clarity in the definition of the free edge. As contrast medium may be retained between the edges of the tear, the hatched area can appear more opaque than the remainder of the meniscus.

producing a shearing strain which the degenerating cartilage is unable to absorb. Such tears are, therefore, commoner in patients after the fourth decade and the injury often appears trivial, e.g. getting up awkwardly from a chair.

Central degeneration implies that the earliest secondary traumatic lesion is a closed tear (Smillie, 1970), and clearly is not demonstrable radiologically or at arthrotomy. As with almost all lesions of the menisci, these are commoner in males and predominantly affect the medial meniscus. They seem to be related to the ageing process and should not be confused with similar tears of the lateral meniscus, which occur in athletic younger males and which have been said to be induced by degeneration. Smillie (1970) uses the terms 'nutritional' and 'cystic' degeneration, respectively, for the old and the young groups.

The finding of a horizontal tear in an elderly subject is not necessarily an indication for active treatment. Chand (1972) found a 63 per cent incidence of tears of the medial meniscus in autopsies on elderly Scottish males without symptoms referable to their knees. Noble and Hamblen (1975) found at least one horizontal tear of a meniscus in 60 per cent of 100 random autopsy examination. Such tears were commoner in medial menisci, larger menisci and in males. Degenerative joint disease was found in 85 per cent of patients in this series.

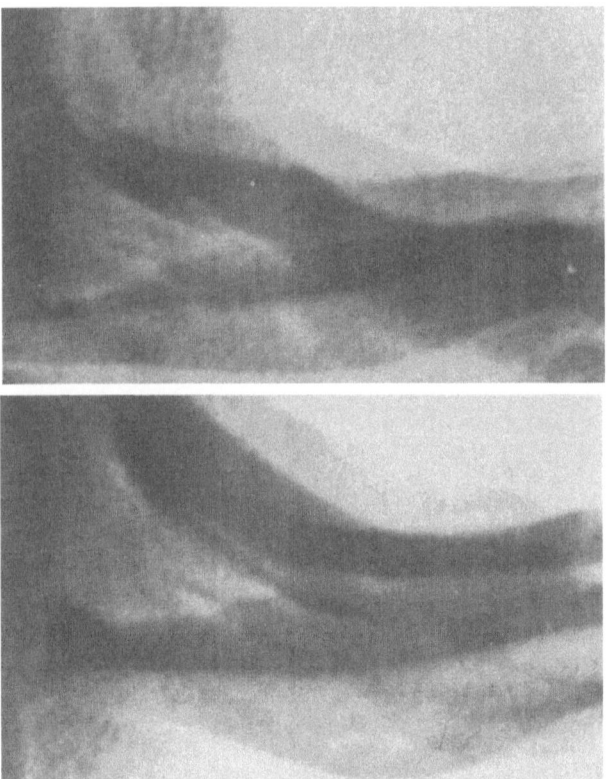

Fig. 6.10 *Horizontal tear of lateral meniscus.* Two views of lateral meniscus showing a horizontal tear involving the inferior surface of the meniscus. Such a lesion would not be directly visible at either arthroscopy or arthrotomy.

Horizontal tears may involve the undersurface of the meniscus (Fig. 6.10) (where they are invisible to the arthoscopist and arthrotomist), the superior surface or at the free edge. Secondary horizontal tears may be demonstrated in the peripheral remnant associated with a vertical tear.

6.2 Peripheral detachment of the menisci

These are dealt with separately because of the differing anatomy of the two menisci. In both, detachments may be complete or incomplete.

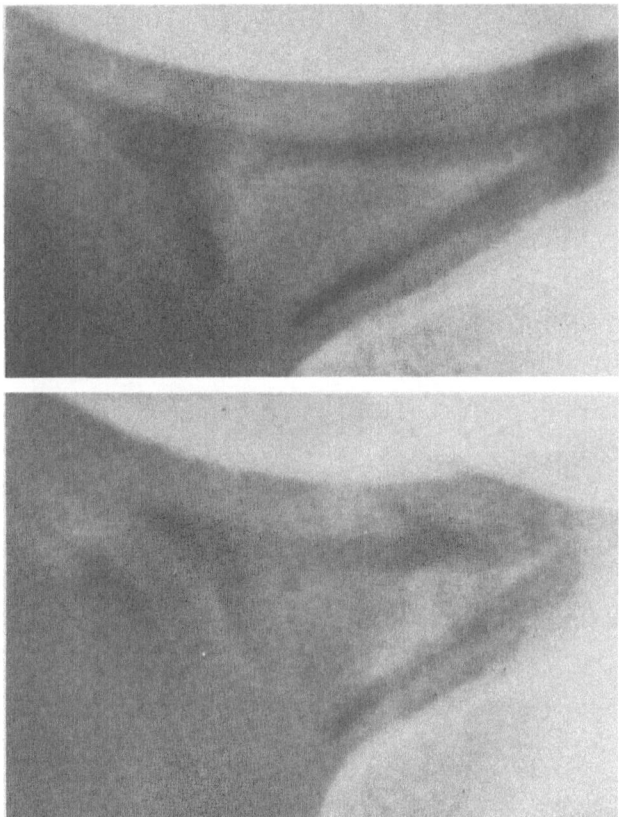

Fig. 6.11 *Peripheral tear of posterior horn of medial meniscus.* Separation of the meniscus has occurred at its superior surface close to the capsular attachment. Such injuries are often associated with haemarthrosis, as they pass through a vascular part of the meniscus. In this patient, a synovitis persisted. Being incomplete, these tears have to be distinguished from large normal recesses; in this case the ragged nature of the defect makes the distinction easy.

In the *medial meniscus*, the appearances do not differ greatly from other vertical tears except, because of the relative bulk at the base of the wedge-like structure, incomplete tears of the superior margin are more common (Fig. 6.11). Such tears transect a vascular region and may be associated with a haemarthrosis. For the

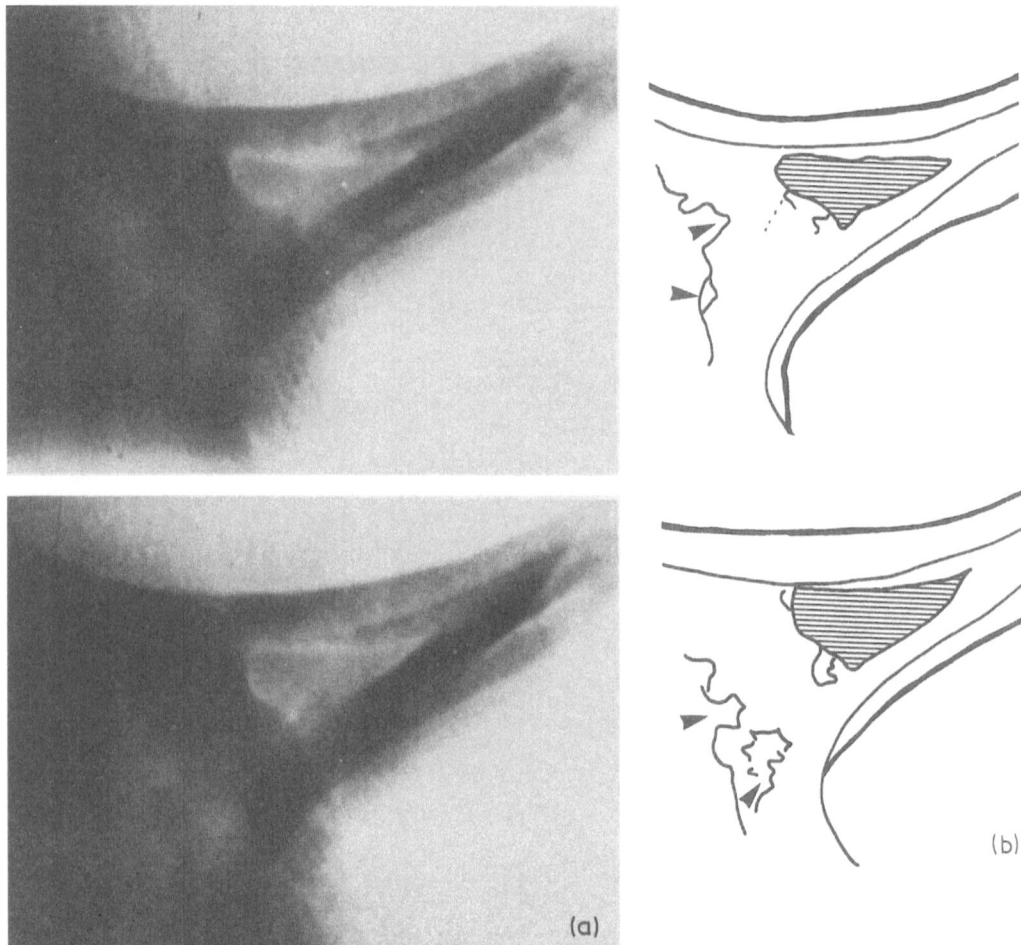

Fig. 6.12 *Complete peripheral detachment of the posterior horn of the lateral meniscus.* (a) The posterior horn is no longer attached by superior and inferior bands to the periphery. The gap between the meniscus and the capsule is abnormally wide, indicating that the detached posterior horn is displaced medially. The irregularities of the peripheral margins (arrowheads) are produced by the torn remnants of the bands. (b) Line drawing of (a).

same reason, healing of the tear can occur, in contrast to tears of the more central avascular parts of the meniscus.

Detachment of the lateral meniscus indicates rupture of one or both of the bands attaching its posterior horn across the popliteus tendon sheath. Complete detachment is self-evident with no bands remaining (Fig. 6.12). Partial detachment

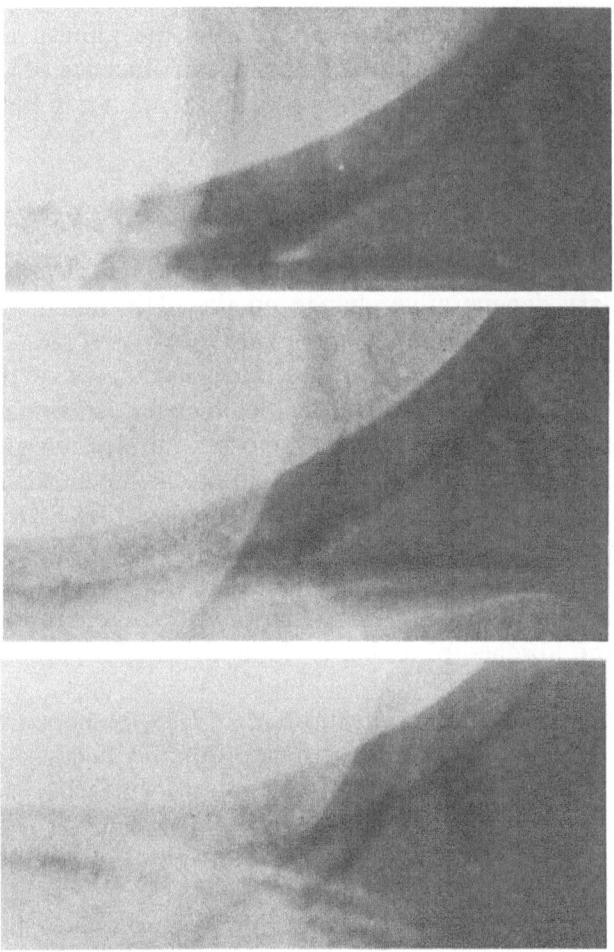

Fig. 6.13 *Probable healed incomplete peripheral tear of posterior horn of medial meniscus.* A deep cleft is present superiorly, causing incomplete separation of the posterior horn. The smooth margins exclude an acute tear; either a healed tear or an abnormally deep recess is the cause. The former seemed the more likely from the arthrographic appearance. Whatever the cause, it seems probable that symptomatic hypermobility could result from such a defect.

is more difficult to establish because of the normal deficiencies relating to the oblique passage of the popliteus tendon sheath (see Chapter 2, page 15).

Individual variation makes the assessment of whether the defect in either band is normal or abnormal difficult indeed. Generally, the tendency is towards underestimation of the defect, leading to false negative errors. Less commonly, the coiled remnant of the detached band can be observed, confirming its disruption.

McIntyre (1972) has described contrast medium escaping from the joint at the point of peripheral detachment of the bands, resulting in loss of radiolucency of the popliteus tendon sheath and, occasionally, demonstration of the tendon and belly of the popliteus muscle by extrasynovial gas.

6.3 Healing and degenerative changes in the meniscus

Apart from evidence of secondary degenerative change on the plain films, it is sometimes possible to determine roughly the age of a meniscal lesion. A recent tear shows sharp or ragged margins. Absorption of contrast into the margin of the meniscus may indicate either the recent nature of the tear or secondary degeneration. An old (over 6 months) tear tends to have smooth rounded margins and, in the case of a peripheral detachment of the medial meniscus, synovial repair produces an appearance which resembles a deep physiological recess (Fig. 6.13).

Healing of incomplete marginal tears can result in the production of tongue-like tags, which are visible on arthrography (Fig. 6.14).

Apart from frank tears of the menisci occurring in association with degeneration, this change may be present in the absence of a clearly defined tear showing the following features:

(a) *absorption of contrast medium* (inbibition – Ricklin *et al.*, 1971). The positive contrast medium permeates the surface of the fibro-cartilage, probably because of surface damage (Fig.6.15). Such damage is commoner on the inferior surface of the meniscus and may be a precursor of early horizontal tears.

(b) *erosion of meniscal surface* indicates repeated minor damage of a type not productive of a rupture ('wear and tear').

(c) *flattening of outline of meniscus*. The meniscus, and this particularly applies to the posterior horn of the medial meniscus, appears to have lost depth, although it remains smooth. It is presumed that this is the effect of sustained pressure on the, now, less elastic fibro-cartilage. Sometimes an appearance resembling meniscectomy is produced (Fig. 6.15).

All these degenerative changes are often associated with changes in the adjoining articular cartilage. Degenerative changes in the menisci are common in the elderly (Noble and Hamblen, 1975) and frequently associated with horizontal cleavage tears. The proportion of troublesome symptoms that can be attributed to degeneration of the meniscus alone is extremely difficult to define.

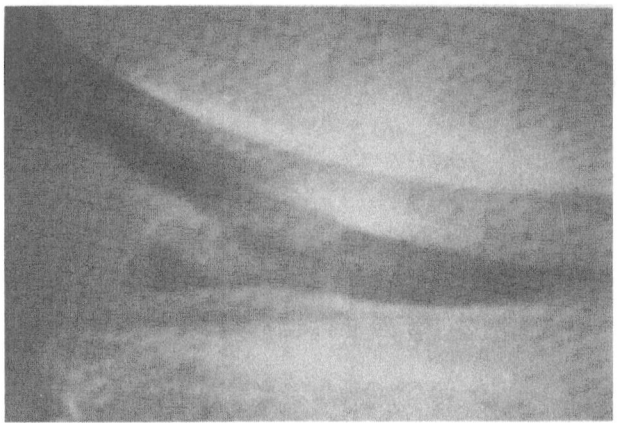

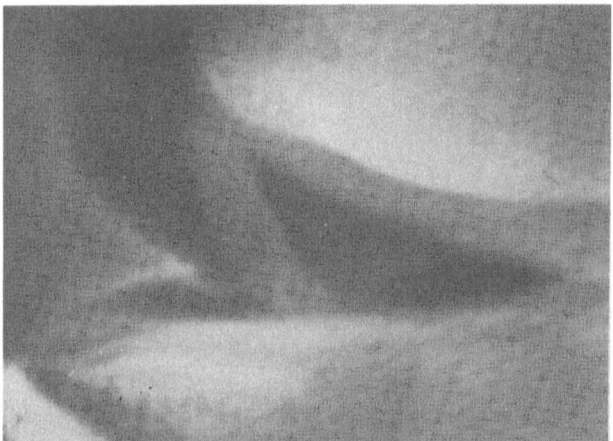

Fig. 6.14 *Tear of medial meniscus*. The patient, a
56-year-old man, had injured his knee a year earlier by
falling down the stairs. The meniscus was shown to be
severely fragmented (top film). The tongue-like
projection (lower film) was observed in relationship to
the anterior half of the meniscus and proved to be a
healed tag, still attached peripherally.

6.4 Post-meniscectomy appearances

Arthrography is requested, not infrequently, because the patient experiences
continued or recurrent symptoms after meniscectomy. Many causes may account
for this situation, e.g. a further lesion of the other meniscus, unconnected ligament
disorders. More often, however, the surgeon wishes to know whether a meniscal
remnant, usually of the posterior horn, has been left behind. The arthrographer

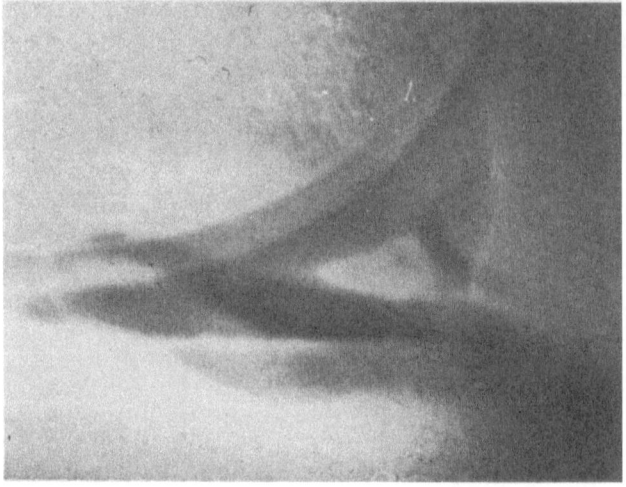

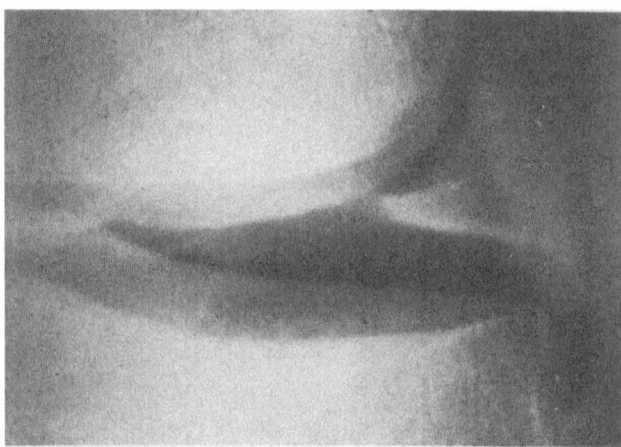

Fig. 6.15 *Damaged posterior horn of lateral meniscus.*
An 18-year-old man with only a 2 month history of
significant trouble in his knee. The arthrogram shows a
small posterior horn of the lateral meniscus with a
blunted free margin into which the medium is
absorbing. These changes of healed trauma resemble
the post-meniscectomy state.

learns by experience what constitutes a reasonable meniscectomy (Fig. 6.16).
Although the meniscus may have been removed almost in its entirity, the increasing
practice of partial meniscectomy (McGinty *et al.*, 1977) naturally leads to a more
variable post-operative appearance and, in our limited experience, to a greater
incidence of subsequent injury to the residual rim or horn of the meniscus, which
has been left behind.

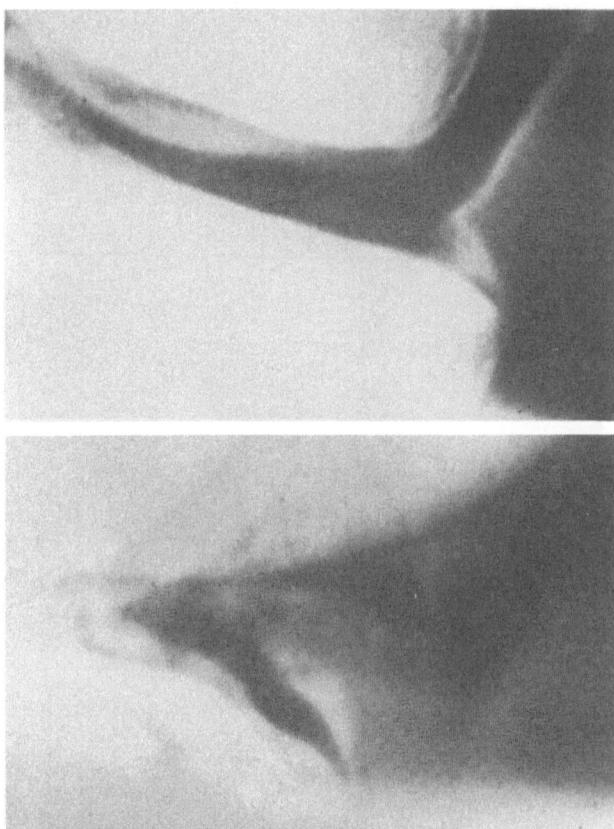

Fig. 6.16 *Post-meniscectomy appearances.* This
45-year-old patient had had a medial meniscectomy
2 years earlier. He gave a history of his knee 'giving
way' for 1 year and a retained posterior horn was
suspected. The arthrogram shows a small and entirely
acceptable remnant of the posterior horn, which was
not responsible for his symptoms; a bucket-handle tear
of his lateral meniscus was demonstrated at the same
arthrogram and was removed surgically.

However, a difference exists between removing the 'handle' of a bucket-handle
tear and attempting a complete meniscectomy and leaving behind the whole, or
most, of the posterior horn of the medial meniscus, sometimes the site of a tear.
Such retained fragments are prone to damage and may be shown to be torn at
arthrography.

Soon after meniscectomy, the residual meniscus shows a ragged margin but, with

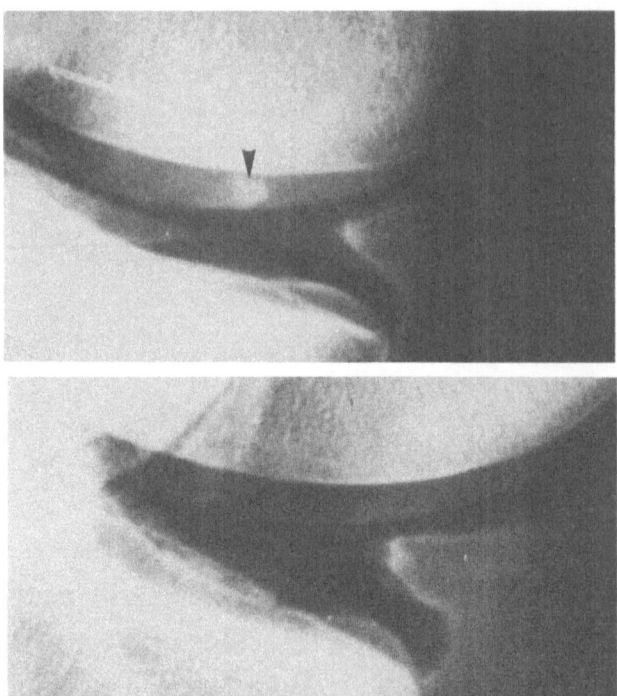

Fig. 6.17 *Post-meniscectomy*. Two views of medial meniscus following a satisfactory meniscectomy. The meniscus is small and shows absorption of contrast medium into its free edge. The posterior horn (lower view) has a slightly irregular margin, but has been adequately removed. The density in the upper picture (arrowed) was considered to be caused by a small loose body.

time, this becomes smooth and rounds off (Fig. 6.17). Its free margin remains blunt. Regeneration of a meniscus, composed of fibrous tissue rather than fibrocartilage, will occur with time. The new meniscus is thinner and smaller than the old and, in my experience, never reaches a cross-sectional area greater than one-third of a normal meniscus. From arthrographic experience, the report of Doyle *et al.* (1966), suggesting that the regenerating meniscus reaches 50 to 60 per cent of its cross-sectional area and that regrowth can be complete in 3 months, seems over-optimistic.

Arthrography can often reveal valuable information in the post-meniscectomy patient, occasionally indicating that the history was erroneous (Fig. 6.18).

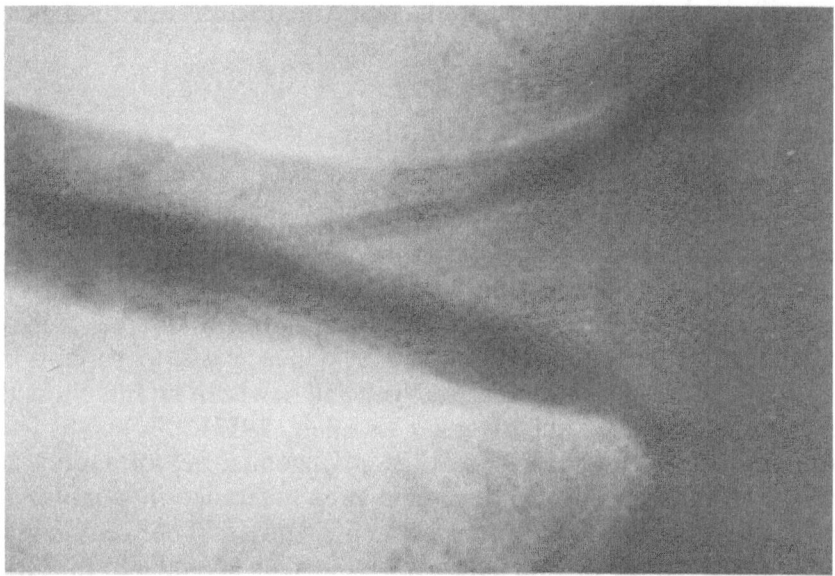

Fig. 6.18 *Tear of posterior horn of medial meniscus.* This patient believed he had had his medial meniscus removed 2 years earlier and arthrography was performed to exclude a large posterior remnant. The arthrographic and operative appearances indicated that, although a previous operation had been performed, the surgeon had decided not to perform a meniscectomy. Although the arthrographic quality is not very satisfactory, the appearances indicate a vertical tear in an otherwise normal meniscus.

6.5 The cystic meniscus

Ganglia or cysts are found primarily in association with the lateral meniscus and are diagnosed clinically by the presence of a lump close to the joint-line, which varies in size with the position of the knee. Such lesions are not demonstrable arthrographic-ally except in the presence of an associated tear, when the cyst may be observed to fill with contrast medium. They are, like ganglia elsewhere, multiloculated and filled with mucinous material. Cysts are found in about 20 per cent of patients at meniscectomy, are rather more common in women than men and are ten times as common in the lateral than the medial meniscus (Raine and Goret, 1972).

Whilst Smillie (1970) believes that the cystic meniscus tends to be confined to young athletic males, Wroblewski (1973), in a series of 500 cystic menisci, has shown that the age of those affected varies from under 10 to over 80 years, with a history of trauma in only 37 per cent. Occasionally, such cystic menisci are bilateral or show an increased familial incidence. Meniscal tears are present in association with about half of the cystic menisci, being rather more common in the presence of a history of injury. Whilst trauma may be one of the factors causing cysts in the menisci, it seems likely that recent injury to the cystic meniscus is usually the cause of the patient presenting to the orthopaedic surgeon.

6.6 Developmental anomalies – the discoid meniscus

A discoid meniscus is one that is thicker and wider than normal and may be attached by the menisco-femoral ligament (Wrisberg) to the medial condyle of the femur. Its posterior horn is not attached to the tibia.

Although it has been suggested that the menisci develop as complete transverse plates, then remodel in the latter half of foetal life, with a discoid meniscus resulting from failure of such remodelling, no evidence exists to support this supposition. In fact, anatomical studies in embryos and newborn infants show that menisci develop in semi-lunar form *ab initio* (Kaplan, 1957).

The discoid meniscus is generally regarded as a congenital malformation. It is found particularly in children and has a female preponderance in symptomatic knees at meniscectomy. Smillie (1970) reported an incidence of 4 per cent in males and 12 per cent in females. The discoid deformity is virtually confined to the lateral meniscus; only a handful of discoid medial menisci are recorded in the literature (Resnick *et al.*, 1976).

The classical association of the 'snapping knee' was first indicated by Kroiss (1910), but these abnormal menisci are also more prone to injury, especially horizontal tears (Ricklin *et al.*, 1971), and Smillie (1970) has suggested that the continuous movement of the femur on the meniscus causes a cleavage lesion of the thickened fibrocartilage.

Evidence in support of the developmental nature of discoid menisci comes from reports of familial incidence (Dashefsky, 1971) and occurrence in both knees (Moës and Munn, 1965). Kaplan (1957) believes the primary defect is the failure of such menisci to be attached to the posterior aspect of the tibial plateau, the menisco-femoral ligament affording an inadequate substitute posteriorly. The meniscus is subject to repeated trauma and becomes secondarily thickened to a discoid shape. Hall (1977) has suggested that at least some discoid lateral menisci could be secondary to a tear of the inferior attaching band of its posterior horn, gradually developing the abnormality in the same way as suggested by Kaplan (1957) in respect of the developmental anomaly. Abnormality or poor visualization of the inferior band in most of Hall's cases could support this contention.

The arthrographic appearance of a completely discoid meniscus is not difficult to interpret, as the meniscus extends centrally towards the intercondylar region, often with parallel surfaces and a bulbous, rather than a triangular, cross-section (Fig.6.19a,b,c).

McIntyre (1972) has emphasized that, at arthrography, the posterior horn of the discoid meniscus fails to rise into the intercondylar notch as a result of its inadequate ligamentous attachment.

Fig. 6.19 *Discoid lateral meniscus.* A 30-year-old male dancer suffered an injury to his left knee. Arthrotomy at another hospital 1 month later revealed no abnormality. After a further 4 months another injury occurred and he was sent for arthrography with a clinical diagnosis of a torn or hypermobile lateral meniscus. Arthrography showed a large meniscus with a small tear of its superior surface. At the subsequent operation, the findings were confirmed and an additional marginal tear was demonstrated. Two views of the meniscus are provided with evidence of a tear in (b), illustrated in the line drawing (c).

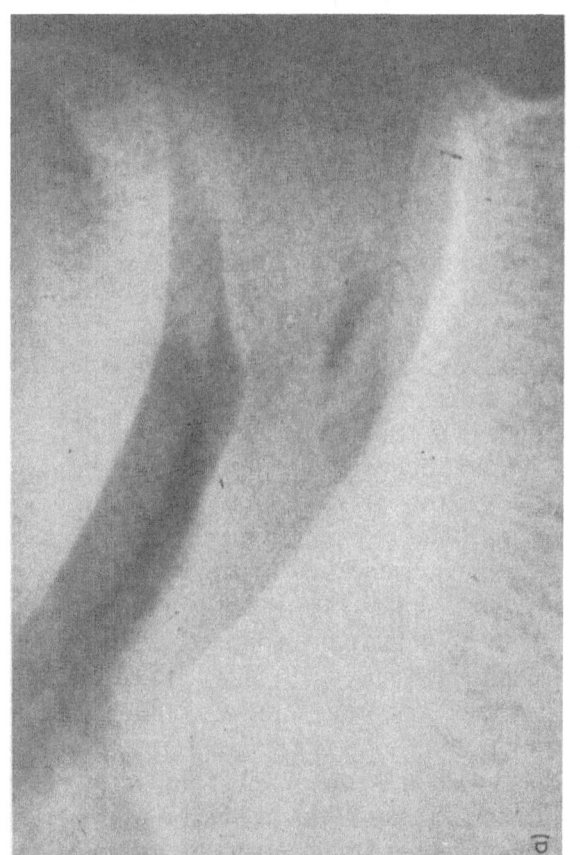

(a)

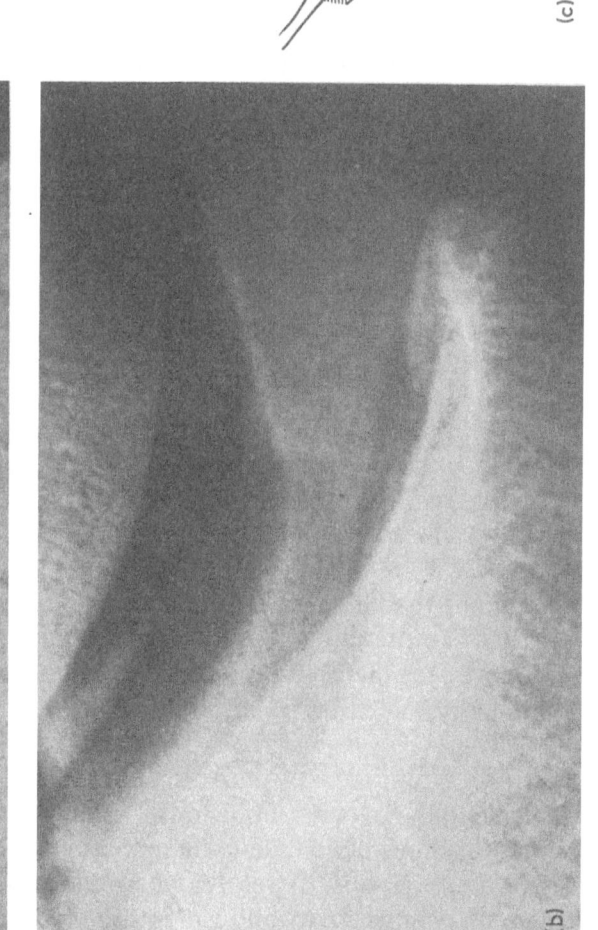

(b)

(c)

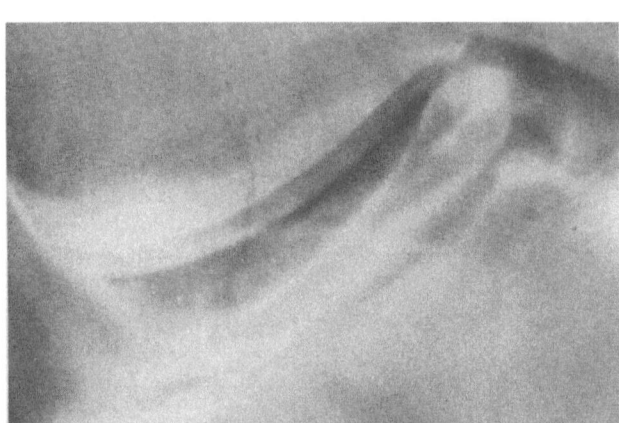

Fig. 6.20 *Discoid lateral meniscus*. The meniscus has lost its normal wedge-shaped cross-section and is a flat plate with a slightly bulbous free edge. The arthrographer finds difficulty in keeping the whole of this type of meniscus in profile.

All discoid menisci are, however, not of the same degree. The arthrographic appearance varies from an almost questionable increase in bulk to a complete disc (Fig. 6.20). In a review of 27 cases of discoid lateral menisci, Hall (1977) described the variation in appearance and defined six types: slab, biconcave, wedge, asymmetric anterior, forme fruste and grossly torn. Whether much is achieved by such complicated typing of a variable feature is doubtful. The forme fruste is most difficult to define, as its indentification depends upon the views of the observer. It has been our practice to call such menisci 'bulky'.

Delineation of the discoid meniscus at arthrography is not always easy. If a meniscus is not in profile, superimposition of the anterior and posterior horn on the middle section may simulate a discoid appearance. This can happen when a patient with a closed meniscal tear resists the stressing of the joint during examination because it is painful. Failure to demonstrate a discoid meniscus may also result from the inability to view the lateral meniscus in profile; the discoid meniscus is, in general, more difficult to manipulate, and the less experienced arthrographer may believe that the absence of a normal profile is due to some error in his technique. Similarly, at arthrography, it is often difficult to demonstrate associated lesions, such as a small parrot-beak tear of the discoid meniscus (Fig. 6.21).

The significance of the discoid meniscus is not always clear, as some are observed incidentally in association with medial compartment symptoms and signs; an increased morbidity due to an increased tendency to tear is undeniable (Fig. 6.22). For these reasons, therefore, where the symptoms and signs indicate a lesion of the lateral compartment and an intact discoid meniscus is shown at arthrography, arthrotomy is advisable. Apart from the morbidity due to the abnormal size, an

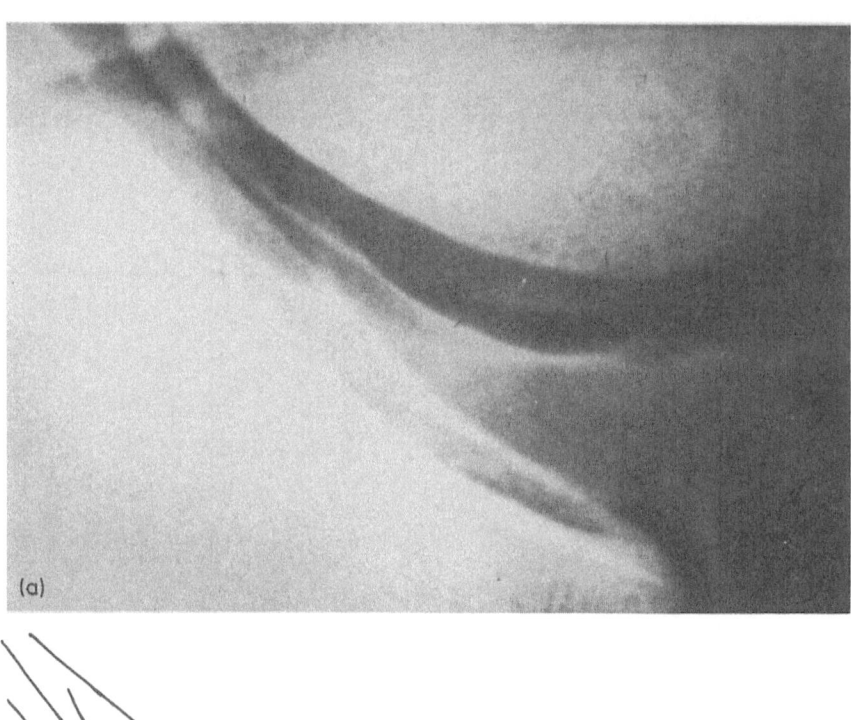

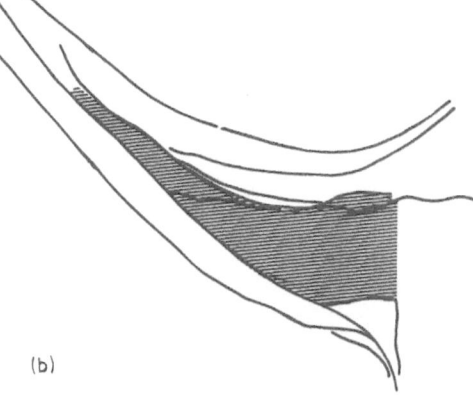

Fig. 6.21 (a) *Parrot-beak tear in partially discoid meniscus.* A 33-year-old woman who gave a 6 year history of retropatellar pain. An initial clinical diagnosis of chondromalacia patellae was questioned when a positive McMurray test suggested a lesion of the lateral meniscus. Arthrography suggested that the meniscus was abnormal and probably torn; a discoid deformity was not noted. At arthroscopy and operation the meniscus was considered to be moderately discoid and showing a small parrot-beak tear. Fibrillation of the articular cartilage of the patella was observed. (b) Line drawing of (a).

increased number of false negative diagnoses of associated tears is to be expected (Hall, 1977).

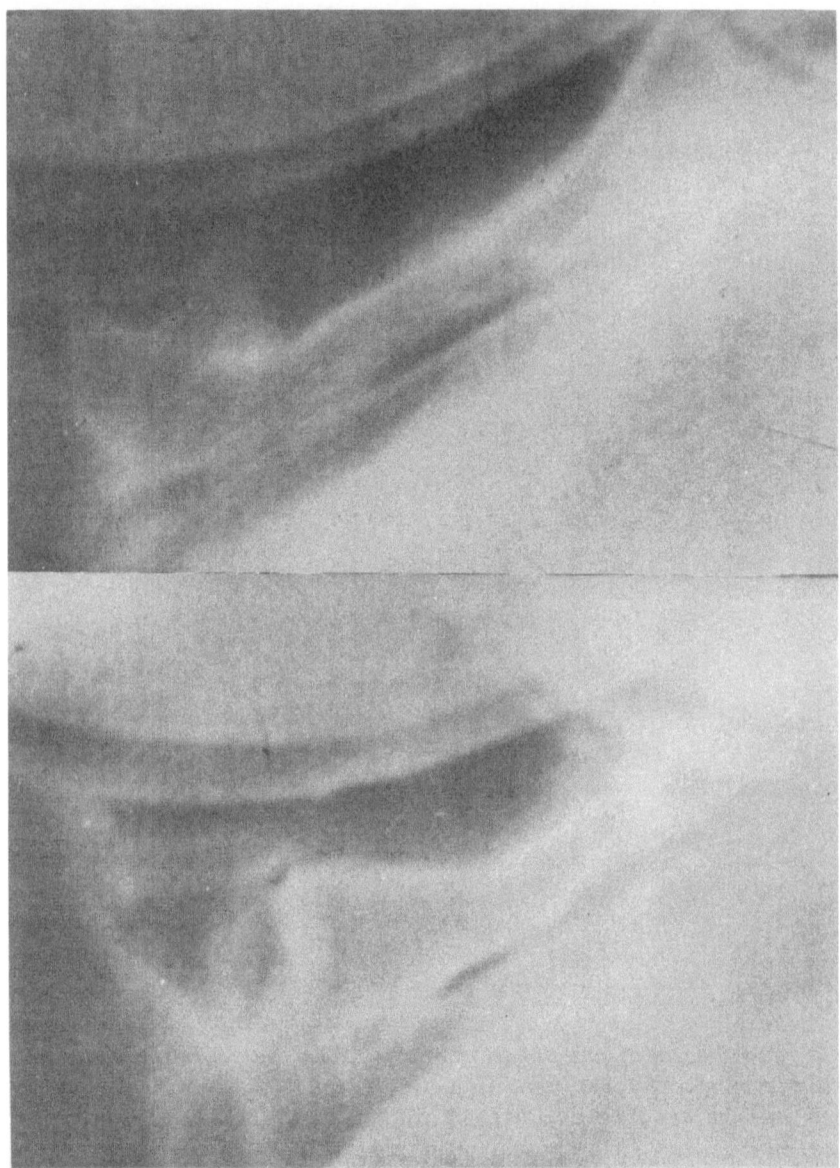

Fig. 6.22 *Tear of posterior horn of medial meniscus.*
Further views of the meniscus shown in Fig. 6.19
demonstrating damage at its peripheral attachment.
Symptomatic discoid menisci often are the site of
complete or incomplete tears.

6.7 Ossification of the meniscus

Demonstration of ossicles within the menisci is uncommon, being first reported by Watson-Jones and Roberts in 1934. Since 1940, a total of 14 cases of menisci containing ossicles have been reported in the English literature, all but one affecting the medial meniscus. Such active bone formation in a fibrocartilaginous body occurs in the usual age group for meniscal disorders, in young male adults with a history of trauma. The aetiology is unknown; it has been suggested that such ossification predisposes to subsequent injury and no report is to be found of an asymptomatic patient with such ossification. These lesions almost always affect the posterior horn of the medial meniscus and are generally misdiagnosed as loose bodies on the plain film: the diagnosis can be confirmed by fluoroscopy (Glass *et al.*, 1975) or arthrography.

6.8 Arthrography of the knee in children

Children constitute a special case and I feel strongly that no operation for meniscectomy in a child should be contemplated before an arthrogram has been performed.

At least two reasons for this view can be put forward:

(a) It is even more important to leave a normal meniscus in a child than in an adult, and only to remove it when evidence of irreparable damage is established. Young children suffer from puzzling internal derangements suggesting locking, but in which a normal meniscus is found (Smillie, 1970).

(b) The incidence of meniscal tears is less in children than in young adults, although the incidence of developmental abnormalities (discoid menisci) is greater.

Stenström (1975) in a series of 600 arthrograms in children found tears in only one-fifth, the youngest being 6 years old. One quarter of all tears were in discoid menisci. The difficulty of the clinical diagnosis of internal derangements of the knee is underlined by the observation that clinical and radiological diagnoses differed in 64 per cent. Operative confirmation of the clinical diagnosis was obtained in only 36 per cent, but in 83 per cent of the radiological diagnoses (90 per cent in respect of meniscal lesions). Similarly, Abrams (1957) in a study covering 10 years in an active orthopaedic hospital for children, discovered true mechanical or developmental lesions of the knees in only seven children under the age of 12 years. In the presence of so few meniscal injuries, it becomes essential that surgical exploration of the child's knee should rarely be undertaken without a preceding arthrogram.

6.9 Recording, reporting and correlating the arthrogram

Whilst the use of a good fluoroscopic apparatus and television chain ensures that most meniscal lesions are visualized in a dynamic way at the time, a permanent record is necessary for the following reasons.

(a) In a minority of cases, the lesion is shown only on the radiograph and, indeed, further supportive views may be required before completing the procedure.

(b) The referring clinician should be offered some confirmation of the abnormality other than the report and, it is suggested, may benefit from some understanding of the radiological anatomy.

(c) When a number of arthrograms are performed at one session, a film record prevents confusion between similar results.

(d) Re-examination of the findings may prove necessary at a future date if discrepancies arise.

6.9.1 Recording

Although video-recording enables the whole examination to be observed at a later

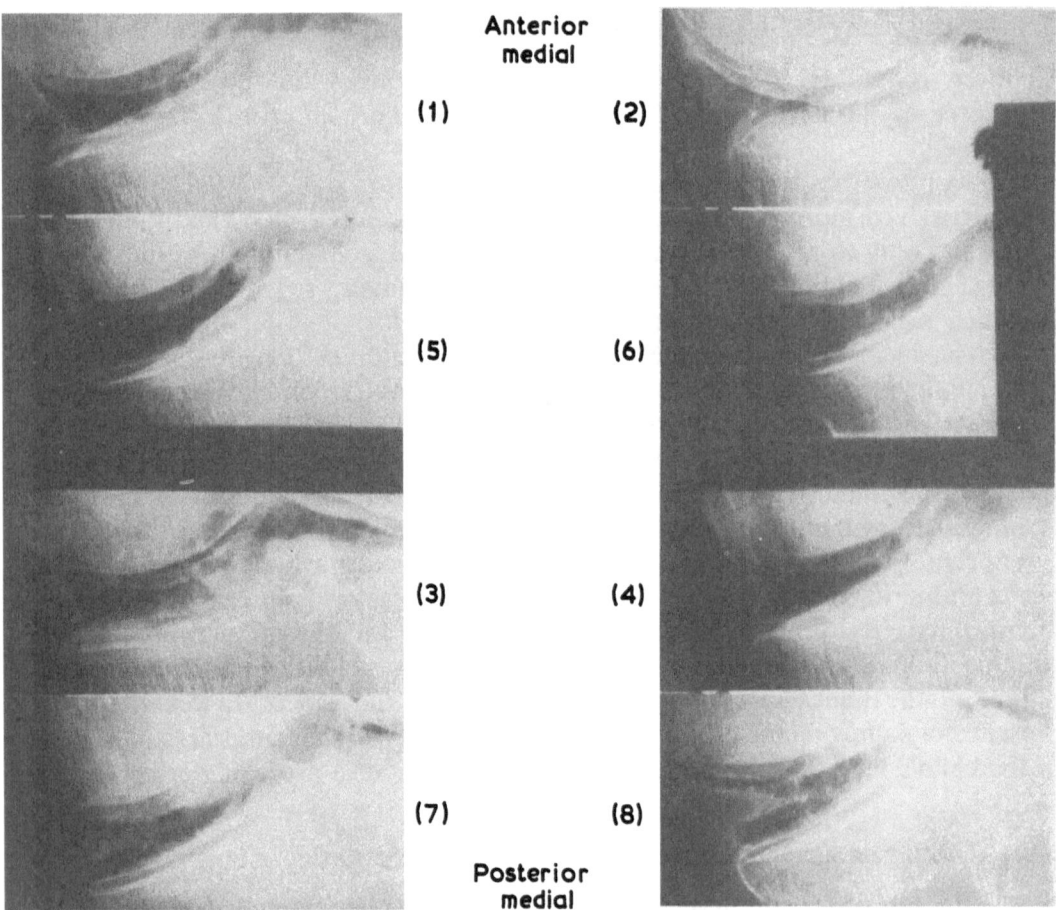

Fig. 6.23 *Recording of arthrogram*. Photograph of film of arthrographic examination of medial meniscus demonstrating eight views on one 24 mm × 30 cm film.

date, it is impractical as a routine record and can be used only for demonstrations or teaching exercises.

6.9.1.1 Conventional radiography

Spot filming of the menisci taken in the optimal positions shown at fluoroscopy remains the best means of recording knee arthrograms. All fluoroscopic apparatus possesses a facility to take small serial films, usually four exposures on a 24 mm × 30 mm film. Certain apparatus is able to record eight small serial exposures on this size of film (Fig. 6.23); the sequence may not be a logical one to the film reader. Using spot films, the radiation to the patient is small, providing the beam is accurately collimated. The radiation received by the radiologist manipulating the patient's foot is also very small, as evidenced by the use of film badges on the operator's finger. The use of lead–rubber gloves is unnecessary.

Radiographic exposures clearly vary with the apparatus used and the film–screen combination. At the present time we employ a 0.3 mm focal spot tube, a focus–subject distance of (very approximately) 70 cm, mammographic film (Agfa-Gevaert) and MR 50 intensifying screens, with radiographic factors of 44 kV, 200 mA, 0.24 s (approx.).

6.9.1.2 70 mm camera and film

Although this technique offers the advantages of speed with reduction in time, cost and radiation dosage, in our experience, the radiographic quality is unacceptable. It may be that better results are obtainable with 100 mm film. In any event, because of the small size of the object, it is important to ensure that electronic magnification of the picture is available (by the provision of two image intensifiers) and the enlarged image can be filmed; in some apparatus the magnification is only available for fluoroscopic viewing.

6.9.1.3 Automatic exposure devices

I have been disappointed by the results obtained with such devices, finding them neither reliable nor reproducible, almost certainly because of the small size of the field. The wide range of densities between cortical bone and gas is another adverse factor. By avoiding the use of these chambers, the radiographer will find it possible to achieve good results by keeping the voltage as low as possible and adjusting the current in the first instance by trial and error. A standard range of exposures can be found, varying the exposure (often only the time element) according to the size of the patient's knee.

6.9.1.4 Film marking

In addition to the normal marking of the film, including the patient's name, the date and the side examined, it is desirable to denote the part of the knee under examination. To this end, all the spot films are viewed from the same side; by convention, each film is displayed as though the patient were facing the observer, e.g. in the right knee the medial meniscus is on the observer's right and the lateral on his left. Each film is then marked ANTERIOR MEDIAL, POSTERIOR MEDIAL, ANTERIOR LATERAL or POSTERIOR LATERAL to indicate the main segments of the menisci. This marking is most conveniently achieved by the use of printed adhesive labels.

Before the completion of the examination, the radiologist determines that the whole of each meniscus has been demonstrated; if not, he will obtain further views. As in all radiological contrast examinations, the format is not stereotyped but should be adapted to circumstances.

6.9.2 Reporting

Radiology is concerned with communication. If the right observation is made, but the wrong description is applied, no credit will be given for the radiological opinion. Many meniscal tears are complex; surgeons view them from their external surface, unlike the radiologist who, by means of serial cross-sections, is enabled to make a more accurate assessment of the direction of the tear. Nevertheless, it is the surgeon with the excised meniscus in his hand who believes he holds the ultimate truth. In reporting, the radiologist should exercise caution until he gains experience. It is wise to state at the outset that the meniscus is either torn or intact, before progressing to a more detailed description of the radiological anatomy of the tear. In this way, the primary conclusion will not be submerged in contradictions over the minutiae in the report.

In the United Kingdom, a period of several months may elapse between arthrography and operation. This time lapse affords an opportunity for a small tear to extend as a result of further injury. Perhaps the most difficult of the common meniscal tears to define clearly at arthrography is the small 'parrot-beak' tear (Fig. 6.21). The meniscus generally appears abnormal or at least suspect, but only experience, resulting from the initial underdiagnosis of such tears, can lead to a greater success in demonstration or definition of the exact form of such a lesion. The other region where experience is particularly necessary is in the assessment of the superior and inferior defects in the bands attaching the posterior horn of the lateral meniscus to the periphery. Careful assessment of the extent of such defects makes all the difference between a normal appearance and a peripheral detachment of the posterior horn.

6.9.3 Correlation of the arthrographic results

The radiologist who is interested in the patient and his problem will demand correlation of his results with the operative findings; such a requirement is not always easy to fulfil. Likewise, he should look down an arthroscope and observe an arthrotomy before talking to the surgeon about the problems that are encountered in the operating theatre. He is then in a position to hold an opinion on the strengths and weaknesses of these diagnostic procedures.

It is helpful to record the results of arthrography together with the initial and final diagnoses and any other relevant data. The use of a simple, but comprehensive duplicated form is advisable. The type used at the Royal National Orthopaedic Hospital is reproduced here (Fig. 6.24). In the recording of results, both surgeons and radiologists should employ line drawings and we include one on our form. Not uncommonly, such drawings correlate better than verbal descriptions; an arthrog-

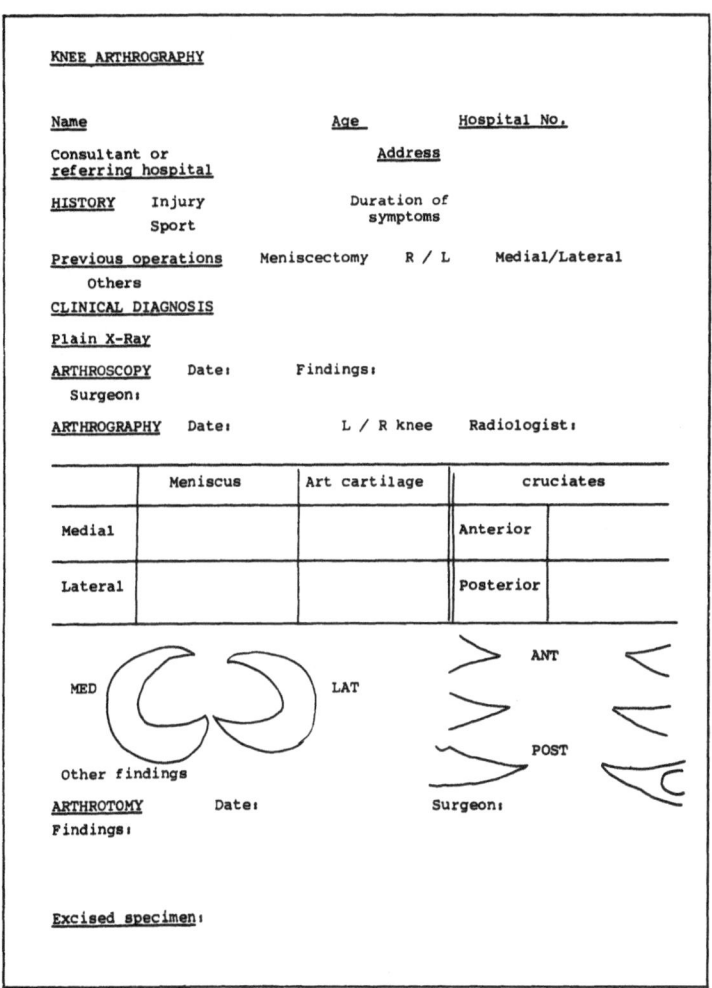

Fig. 6.24 *Record of investigatory procedures.* An example of a form for recording the findings at arthrography, arthroscopy and operation.

raphic description of a 'frayed margin with absorption of contrast medium into the free edge' may prove to be identical in practice to the surgeon's 'degenerate meniscus with incomplete marginal tears'. Although, theoretically, the excised meniscus offers the most acceptable final demonstration of its state, this too is not beyond dispute. A meniscus which is the site of a detached bucket-handle tear may have its detached margin either lying beside the rim or displaced centrally into the intercondylar region, resulting in a different disposition at the time of arthrography/ arthroscopy. Removal of a meniscus may cause it to tear or the meniscectomy incision may extend into a posterior horn tear, giving the surgeon no evidence of the earlier injury from the excised specimen. Occasions will occur when the radiologist has a better view of the meniscus than the surgeon and is, therefore, more likely to be correct in his assessment. It must be emphasized that the surgeon can only justify his final diagnosis when his visualization of the suspect region is complete.

References

Abrams, R.C. (1957). Meniscus lesions of the knee in young children. *Journal of Bone and Joint Surgery*, **39–A**, 194–5.

Chand, K. (1972). Horizontal (cleavage) tears of the knee joint menisci in the elderly. *Journal of the American Geriatrics Society*, **20**, 430–3.

Dalinka, M.K., Coren, G.S. and Wershba, M. (1973). Knee arthrography. *CRC Critical Reviews in Clinical Radiology and Nuclear Medicine, 4*, 1–59.

Dashefsky, J.H. (1971). Discoid lateral meniscus in three members of a family. *Journal of Bone and Joint Surgery*, **53–A**, 1208–10.

Doyle, J.R., Eisenberg, J.H. and Orth, M.W. (1966). Regeneration of knee menisci: a preliminary report. *Journal of Trauma*, **6**, 50–5.

Glass, R.S., Barnes, W.M., Kells, D.U., Thomas, S. and Campbell, C. (1975). Ossicles of knee menisci. Report of seven cases. *Clinical Orthopedics, 111*, 163–71.

Hall, F.M. (1977). Arthrography of the discoid lateral meniscus. *American Journal of Roentgenology*, **128**, 993–1002.

Kaplan, E.B. (1957). Discoid lateral meniscus of the knee joint. Nature mechanism and operative treatment. *Journal of Bone and Joint Surgery*, **39–A**, 77–87.

Kroiss, F. (1910). Die Verletzungen der Kniegelenks-zwischenknorpel und ihrer Verbindungen. *Beiträge zur Klinischen Chirurgie Tübing*, **66**, 598–801.

McGinty, J.B., Geuss, L. F. and Marvin, R.A. (1977). Partial or total meniscectomy. *Journal of Bone and Joint Surgery*, **59–A**, 763–6.

McIntyre, J.L. (1972). Arthrography of the lateral meniscus. *Radiology*, **105**, 531–6.

Moës, C.A. and Munn, J.D. (1965). The value of knee arthrography in children. *Journal of Canadian Association of Radiologists, 16*, 226–33.

Nicholas, J.A., Freiberger, R.H. and Killoran, P.J. (1970). Double-contrast arthrography of the knee. Its value in the management of 225 knee derangements. *Journal of Bone and Joint Surgery*, **52–A**, 203–20.

Noble, J. and Hamblen, D.L. (1975). The pathology of the degenerate meniscus lesion. *Journal of Bone and Joint Surgery*, **57–B**, 180–6.

Raine, G.E. and Gonet, L.C. (1972). Cysts of the menisci of the knee. *Postgraduate Medical Journal*, **48**, 49–51.

Resnick, D., Goergen, T.G., Kaye, J.J., Ghelman, B. and Wood, P.R. (1976). Discoid medial meniscus. *Radiology*, **121**, 575–6.

Ricklin, P., Rüttimann, A. and Del Buono, M.S. (1971). *Meniscus Lesions*. Georg Thieme Verlag, Stuttgart.

Smillie, I.S. (1970). *Injuries of the Knee Joint* 4th Edn. Livingstone, Edinburgh.

Stenström, R. (1975). Diagnostic arthrography of traumatic lesions of the knee joint in children. *Annales de Radiologie, Paris*, **18**, 391–4.

Watson-Jones, R. and Roberts, R.E. (1934). Calcification, decalcification and ossification. *British Journal of Surgery*, **21**, 461–99.

Wroblewski, B.M. (1973). Trauma and the cystic meniscus: Review of 500 cases. *Injury*, **4**, 319–21.

7 Accuracy, results, sources of diagnostic error: Illustrative cases

7.1 Accuracy

Numerous published studies have shown that, in experienced hands and employing a careful technique, arthrography can achieve an accuracy in excess of 90 per cent in the diagnosis of meniscal injuries (Freiberger *et al.*, 1966, Kiss and Moir, 1968, Butt and McIntyre, 1969; Brown *et al.*, 1978, Thijn, 1979).

The accuracy of clinical diagnosis in some series has also been as high (Smillie, 1970). Nevertheless, an increasing awareness of the limitations of the clinical signs of meniscal damage has led to the introduction of the investigative techniques of arthrography and arthroscopy. Despite the irrefutable evidence that arthrography can be a highly accurate investigation, each radiologist will wish to determine the accuracy of his own technique, because it is this that is of major interest to his surgical colleagues. A high degree of accuracy cannot be expected immediately. Even when the technical problems are controlled so that a reproducible examination can be expected, experience must be gained in the interpretation of arthrograms. This takes time, because it requires the examination of scores of arthrograms to establish the normal and the common deviations from the normal resulting from minor injuries of the menisci.

7.1.1 Results

In the assessment of the accuracy of any diagnostic procedure, a generally accepted criterion for the definitive diagnosis is required. In many diseases, histological examination provides the final and presumably correct diagnosis. In disorders of the menisci, it has been accepted in the past that the diagnosis is established at operation. As currently practised on the knee joint, however, arthrotomy has certain shortcomings.

(a) The small operative field of vision often does not permit complete visualization of the meniscus and this particularly applies to the posterior horn of the medial meniscus – the part most commonly injured.

(b) An injury may only be demonstrated when the meniscus is removed.

(c) Of greater concern is the possibility of removing a damaged meniscus in such a way that the incision made by the meniscotome extends in continuity into a tear of the posterior horn, so that the tear remains totally undiagnosed.

(d) The need to examine the posterior horn directly or indirectly with a probe or hook, to determine whether the meniscus is abnormal *in situ* is not always appreciated. When taken in combination with (c) above, it is possible for meniscal lesions to be missed completely.

(e) Conversely, a normal meniscus may be torn during removal and the damage attributed to a previous injury. Because of the limitation of direct visualization of the posterior horn of the meniscus at arthrotomy, it has been our practice, when reporting a tear confined to the posterior horn of the medial meniscus, to advise the surgeon to test the peripheral attachment of the meniscus with a hook or similar instrument. In this way, it is usually possible to establish the presence of an abnormality before undertaking meniscectomy; this is not an attempt to teach the surgeon his job, but to draw his attention to the exact anatomical location of the tear as observed by the radiologist. As a consequence, when diagnostic doubt exists, the information most likely to be correct in any specific case should be accepted; if no diagnostic procedure is entirely satisfactory, the diagnosis cannot be established. Thus, when a technically satisfactory arthrogram shows a tear of the posterior horn of the medial meniscus and the arthroscopic examination is normal, but does not demonstrate the posterior horn, the arthrographic findings are likely to be correct. When the arthrogram is poor, perhaps as a result of synovitis, and the arthroscopy shows a parrot-beak tear of the lateral meniscus, which is not confirmed at operation as the meniscus was fragmented at removal, the arthroscopic findings are the ones most likely to be correct.

Much stress is rightly laid on the incidence of positive and negative diagnostic errors in any diagnostic technique, the point being that, although a negative error is undesirable, a positive error results often in the removal of a normal meniscus. Nevertheless, the overall importance of any investigation is reflected in its effect on the management of the patient; in this respect, the demonstration of a normal meniscus in a patient referred with a suspected meniscal tear must be one of the more valuable findings, although often given little emphasis in many series. The details of the first 1000 arthrograms undertaken by our department are shown in Table 7.1, which has been divided into two parts; (a) relates to 835 patients who had not undergone meniscectomy and (b) to the 165 patients who had had a previous meniscectomy. In (a), 416 of the 835 arthrograms (or almost exactly 50 per cent) were found to show normal menisci.

The presence of a clinical diagnosis of a meniscal tear suggests that, without the use of arthrography or arthroscopy, at least some of this group would have been subjected to an exploratory operation. In fact, even after a normal arthrographic examination, in our series, this finding was ignored in 37 patients who were

Table 7.1 Results of 1000 arthrograms

(a) 835 arthrograms prior to surgery

Radiological findings	Operative findings				
	Normal	Tear of medial meniscus	Tear of lateral meniscus	Degeneration	No operation
Normal	37	8	12	2	357
Tear of medial meniscus	19	163	0	5	56
Tear of discoid lateral menisus	2	0	53	2	14
Degeneration of meniscus	3	7	4	19	72

(b) 165 arthrograms following meniscectomy

Radiological findings	Operative findings					
	Adequate meniscectomy	Large remnant	Tear of remnant	Other meniscus torn	Other meniscus degenerate	No further operation
Adequate meniscectomy	15	0	0	5	0	71
Large meniscal remnant	0	18	0	0	0	19
Tear of meniscal remnant	0	1	5	0	0	2
Tear of other meniscus	2	0	0	17	2	5
Other meniscus degenerate	0	0	0	2	0	1

subjected to arthrotomy and shown to have no meniscal abnormality. Although the clinician must always retain the right to manage his case in accordance with the overall results of investigation, even to the extent of conducting a diagnostic arthrotomy, these 37, perhaps unnecessary, operations exceeded the number of radiological false positive examinations.

Examination of the radiological errors in more detail is shown in Tables 7.2 and 7.3. These gross figures are gleaned from operative conclusions.

In the *false negative* group, eight medial meniscal tears were apparently not visualized at arthrography. In most of these the error was one of interpretation by the arthrographer, sometimes contributed to by a poor examination due to synovitis; in three cases, the meniscal tear was missed in the presence of another abnormality correctly diagnosed (loose bodies on two occasions and a lateral meniscal tear once). Twelve tears of the lateral meniscus were missed; three others

Table 7.2 Analysis of false negative arthrographic results based on operative conclusions

Arthrographic findings	Operation			
Medial meniscal tears (8)	Tear posterior horn	Parrot-beak tear	Loose body + tear	
No meniscal tear	5	—	—	
Lateral meniscal tear, medial meniscus intact	1	—	—	
Loose body, no meniscal tear	—	1	1	
Lateral meniscal tears (12)	Major tear	Radial tear	Detached posterior horn	Small parrot-beak tear
Meniscus intact	6*	1	2	3
Degenerative menisci (2)				

*In three of these, operation was carried out after an interval of between 5 months and 3 years of arthrography; two of these patients sustained further injuries in the interval.

Table 7.3 Analysis of false positive arthrographic results based on operative conclusions

Arthrographic findings	Operation		
	No tear	Loose body only	Operative view inadequate or suspect
Medial meniscal tears (19)			
Complete posterior horn tear	—	2	11
Incomplete posterior horn tear	1 (deep sulcus)	—	—
Anterior horn tear	1*	—	—
Horizontal tear	1	—	—
Meniscal tear + loose bodies	—	1	—
Tear suspected only	2	—	—
Lateral meniscal tears (2) 1 small posterior horn tear 1 incomplete posterior horn tear	} Neither confirmed at operation		
Degenerative menisci (3)			
Normal	Reported as thin not degenerative		Operative view inadequate
1	1		1

*Mobile anterior horn of meniscus + pedunculated synovial fold.

had been operated upon from 5 months to 3 years after arthrography and two of these had a clear history of further injury.

In the *false positive* group, although 19 medial meniscal tears shown at arthrography were not confirmed at operation, in 11 of these the operative findings were unacceptable for a conclusive diagnosis. In the majoriy of these, the posterior horn (which was the site of the tear described) was not visualized and the surgeon was in no position to claim that it was normal. Such phrases as 'anterior two-thirds of meniscus appeared normal' and 'if this meniscus is torn then it is only a detached posterior horn' indicate that the radiologist obtains a better view of the posterior horn under these circumstances.

In the lateral meniscus, two small tears of the posterior horn were diagnosed at arthrography but not confirmed at operation.

In order to assess the percentage accuracy or error, it is necessary to know the final diagnosis of the cases in each group. As the arthrographic diagnosis of a normal meniscus should generally not lead to an operation, it is not possible to establish a final diagnosis in the majority of the false negative cases. Obviously, it might be possible by long-term surveillance to determine whether patients' symptoms and signs settled or persisted; we did not find this a practicable proposition, feeling that, even at the end of a clinical surveillance, a final diagnosis might not be forthcoming.

In respect of the incidence of false positive diagnoses, the situation is more acceptable. Only those arthrotomies where the surgeon had actually visualized the meniscal tear were included, leaving a total of 176 patients with an arthrographic diagnosis of a tear of the medial meniscus. Tears were demonstrated surgically in 163, giving an accuracy for arthrography of 92.6 per cent. If the five menisci, described as tears and shown at operation to be degenerative, are included as overall meniscal lesions, the accuracy rises to 95.5 per cent for the medial meniscus – a false positive error of 4.5 per cent.

7.2 Arthrography and arthroscopy

It is perhaps unfortunate that a tendency exists for promotion of the advantages and accuracy of one of these techiques to the exclusion of the other. Both have their advantages and disadvantages and the arthrographer who diagnoses a minor meniscal tear or who produces a non-diagnostic examination for technical reasons should not hesitate to suggest that arthroscopy be performed as a next essential step towards obtaining a correct diagnosis. Similarly, if the arthroscopist does not visualize the suspect region to his satisfaction, arthrography should be recommended. The comparison of the results of an experienced arthroscopist with those of an inexperienced arthrographer (Jackson and Abe, 1972) or vice versa, is a valueless exercise. For this reason, it is essential that the two procedures, when practised in the same hospital, are supervised or performed by those with experience in each method, so that it is possible to compare like with like. We have been fortunate in our hospital for this to have been the case for many years.

7.3 Results of arthrography and arthroscopy

In 160 cases arthroscopy was performed. In 50 of these the arthroscopic findings agreed with those of arthrography and were confirmed at operation. It is interesting to note that at three of the operations no meniscal abnormality was at first observed. Further exploration, which revealed a meniscal tear, was prompted by the findings of the preceding diagnostic procedures.

In 53 cases the arthroscopic and arthrographic findings were in agreement, but operation was not performed; many of these patients showed no evidence of a meniscal lesion.

In three cases, arthrography and arthroscopy were agreed on the presence of an abnormality, but operative findings differed. In one, an abnormal anterior horn of the medial meniscus was interpreted by the surgeon at exploration as a pedunculated synovial fold, which was excised. In another, a tag arising from the posterior horn of the lateral meniscus was found to be a loose body in relation to an intact meniscus. In a third case, both arthroscopy and arthrography demonstrated an abnormality of the posterior horn of the medial meniscus, but neither actually showed the meniscal tear that was apparent at operation.

In 16 cases, the arthrographic findings did not agree with arthroscopy and operation. In three patients, the error was partial or a change had occurred. One patient was diagnosed arthrographically as having a probable small tear of the medial meniscus; at operation, 3 months later, this was shown to be a bucket-handle tear. Another, reported as normal, was found to have a bucket-handle tear of the lateral meniscus; in the interval of 5 months between the two examinations, the patient had received a number of further injuries to the knee and the symptom of locking had appeared. The third patient was reported at arthrography as having a suspect medial meniscus; a parrot-beak tear was found at operation. The remaining 13 arthrographic errors were:

(1) arthrography failed to diagnose three medial meniscal tears – two of these were small and, in the third (early in the series) the patient had considerable synovitis, which probably caused the error;

(2) one suspected medial meniscal tear was not confirmed;

(3) one diagnosed medial meniscal tear was not confirmed;

(4) six lateral menisci were diagnosed as normal and tears were subsequently found, four of these were parrot-beak tears. Another was a posterior horn detachment, whilst the last was an extensive tear found at operation 4 months after arthrography. In two further patients diagnosed at arthrography as degenerate and discoid lateral menisci, respectively, tears were shown at operation.

In 14 patients, arthroscopic errors occurred, none of these was a false positive result. In 13 of the cases, arthroscopy failed to diagnose tears of the medial meniscus, the tear being predominantly of the posterior horn in ten of the knees. In one patient, the examination failed to demonstrate a tear of the lateral meniscus.

In the remainder of the series discrepancies occurred; arthrography and arthroscopy failed to agree in 16 cases where no operative correlation was obtained. In most of these, gross abnormality was not suspected by either diagnostic method.

In five cases, arthrography demonstrated a tear of the medial meniscus, which was not shown at arthroscopy or operation. These have not been included in the earlier groups, as the latter two examinations failed to demonstrate the region (posterior horn) where the tear was suspected.

In the final few cases, no correlation was obtained between any of the three investigatory procedures.

An analysis of the results is presented in Table 7.4. Because some doubt

Table 7.4 Results of arthroscopy and arthrography – 160 patients

	No. patients	%
Arthrography, arthroscopy and operation agree	50	31
Arthrography and arthroscopy agree, no operation	53	33
Arthrographic findings did not agree with arthroscopy or operation	16	10
Arthroscopic findings did not agree with arthrography or operation	14	9
Operation not in agreement with other two investigations	3	2
Arthrography and arthroscopy disagree. No operation	16	10
Arthrography diagnosed meniscus lesion, but suspect region not visualized at arthroscopy or operation	5	3
No real correlation	3	2
	160	100

inevitably must exist in those cases where a final diagnosis was not established, Table 7.5 shows the results in 137 cases where this was not the case. These figures indicate that the two examinations have a similar accuracy in the diagnosis of meniscal injuries.

Table 7.5 Comparison between arthrography and arthroscopy in 137 patients where the final diagnosis was not disputed.

	Arrthrography		Arthroscopy	
Correct	118 ⎫		120 ⎫	
	⎬ (89.8%)		⎬ (88.3%)	
Incompletely correct	5 ⎭		1 ⎭	
False positive result	4	(2.9%)	2	(1.5%)
False negative results	10	(7.3%)	14	(10.2%)

Certain conclusions can probably be made in the comparison between arthrography and arthroscopy from these results:

(1) The two methods show similar numbers of errors and an equally high level of accuracy.

(2) Arthroscopy rarely produces false positive results; the majority of errors stem from failure to visualize the posterior horn of the meniscus, hence posterior horn tears, particularly of the medial meniscus, are missed.

(3) Unlike arthroscopy, arthrography may not always be performed in the period immediately prior to operation. Whilst a few weeks delay is unlikely to alter the picture, in a period of 5 to 6 months before operation, further damage is certainly possible as several patients' histories indicate.

(4) Most errors of arthrography are those of technique or interpretation. Sometimes a non-diagnostic examination is achieved as a result of synovitis or some other complication at the time.

(5) Arthrographic errors commonly occur with the smaller tears and, in this group of patients which was also arthroscoped, the radial or parrot-beak tears predominated, errors being more common on the lateral side.

7.4 Sources of diagnostic error

Nothing makes up for experience, and particularly rewarding is the experience of one's own mistakes. In this chapter, it is intended to concentrate on errors of technique and interpretaion. It must be emphasized that there is no such thing as a standard arthrogram. The patient's examination is not complete until all the films have been inspected and any further views taken if required.

Certain areas of the examination give more than their fair share of problems and these will be discussed.

As in all radiological practice, it will be found that the majority of errors are caused by two sets of circumstances:

(1) failure to observe a radiological feature or, if observed, failure to apply the correct interpretation;

(2) acceptance of an examination, which is technically inadequate for a variety of reasons.

Human nature cannot be altered and errors of perception will continue to be made. One can hope to minimize incorrect interpretation and, in this chapter, the reader's attention is directed to areas where problems are most likely to arise.

7.4.1 The anterior horn

It is not our experience that tears of the anterior horn are very common. Smillie (1970) found tears of the anterior horn in only 100 of 4500 meniscectomies. The warning by Dalinka et al. (1973) that these tears are frequently overlooked may indicate that we are missing the lesions, but only rarely are we shown an excised meniscus with a tear of the anterior horn, undiagnosed before operation.

Hall (1976) has commented on the difficulties experienced in determining the integrity of the anterior horn of either meniscus as the lateral projection is approached; this results from the small size of this part of the normal meniscus, which often does not possess a clean triangular cross-section, and the overlapping shadows of other synovial structures.

Most of the troublesome images are caused by synovial reflections from the infrapatellar fat pad (Ricklin et al., 1971), which is variable in size and shape and therefore leads to an infinite variation of synovial folds. In addition, the tongue-shaped projection of the synovial-covered fat pad itself can overlie the meniscus and simulate a tear (Ricklin et al., 1971).

More posteriorly in the anterior horn, as the meniscus enlarges, the margin of its smaller anterior portion overlies the anterolateral part under study and may simulate a tear. In both these situations caution in the interpretation is advisable, so that tears are not erroneously diagnosed in the presence of a small, somewhat irregular, yet normal anterior horn; further views are obtained to establish that such overlying features are not in the same plane as the part under examination.

The section of the lateral meniscus between the anterior horn and the upward emergence of the popliteus tendon sheath is perhaps the meniscal region least amenable to full double-contrast display. This is probably due to its loose peripheral attachments but, whatever the cause, the meniscus tends to float upwards, seeming to be loosely adherent to the femoral condyle. An orthograde projection frequently requires flexion of the knee; failure to achieve this may result in the suggestion of a tear or, more probably, a pseudo-discoid appearance. Further views in varying degrees of flexion should be obtained if any doubt persists.

7.4.2 Peripheral detachments

Peripheral detachments may be simulated on the lateral side by the normal relationships of the popliteus rendon sheath, on the medial side by large recesses and the overlying gastrocnemio-semimembranosus bursa and on both sides by contrast medium in the pericapsular tissues.

7.4.2.1 Lateral meniscus

Only a sound knowledge of the normal anatomy and arthrographic appearance can give any confidence in the assessment of the peripheral attachments of the lateral meniscus. Even then, the differentiation between minor detachments of the bands and normal variation can be extremely speculative. In all reported series, this area accounts for most negative errors. It is right that this should remain the case, for to increase accuracy to the level achieved with medial meniscus tears would certainly risk the removal of some normal lateral menisci.

7.4.2.2 Medial meniscus

Both shallow superior recesses (Hall, 1976) (Fig. 5.2c) and overlying bursae can simulate surface tears. The bursal image can also give the impression of a vertical tear, but like many other overlying contrast-filled structures, not only does the 'tear' not contain air as well as positive-contrast medium, but it does not bear a constant relationship to the meniscus.

Deep recesses often simulate healed peripheral tears and it is sometimes impossible to determine which is present. As any defect of this depth, from whatever cause, can produce hypermobility, argument is probably immaterial and any further action should be taken on grounds of clinical disability.

Ricklin et al.(1971) have suggested classification into well-rounded, smooth recesses and large, uneven, suspect recesses. This does not completely solve the problem of the smooth, healed peripheral tear (Fig. 6.13).

It is not uncommon for contrast medium, usually gas, either to be injected extra-articularly or to escape from the joint at some stage of the examination. The extent and peripheral location of the lucent linear shadow should prevent its being mistaken for a tear.

7.4.3 Marginal irregularities

Hall (1976) has demonstrated a lesion which he believes is due to a localized tear of the coronary ligament of the posterior horns of the medial meniscus. Such nipple-like prominences are seen from time to time and could well be the result of healed coronary ligament tears. It is not yet established that such tears extend to produce peripheral detachment of the posterior horn. Fortunately, the course of such injuries has been assumed to be towards healing and conservative management is recommended.

7.4.4 Variations in the size and shape of the meniscus

The *size* of the meniscus in the presence of an otherwise normal appearance is not necessarily abnormal, particularly if the normal triangular cross-section is preserved. It is usual for the menisci on both sides of the joint to be of comparable size and they then can be assumed to be normal. Undoubtedly, on occasions, an alteration in the size of one meniscus can be the result of trauma, but the radiologist should be cautious before he suggests this possibility. However, a localized reduction in size in one part of a meniscus is usually abnormal and due to the detachment of a fragment of meniscus. This is rarely achieved without alteration in shape.

Any departure from the normal meniscal *shape* must be regarded with great suspicion. Such changes include the loss of a triangular cross-section, absence of a smooth meniscal surface and blunting of the normal sharp margin of the meniscus.

Particular care must be taken in the case of the posterior half of the medial meniscus. The posterior horn normally has a concave upper surface and a convex inferior surface (Fig. 5.2c). Sometimes a portion of the posterior horn of the meniscus is detached, usually from its under-surface, resulting in a meniscal outline on arthrography which is either an equilateral triangle or shows a concavity of its under-surface.

As the posterior horn of the medial meniscus has the largest cross-sectional area of any part of either meniscus, such an alteration in shape is accompanied by some reduction in size, so that the posterior horn appears no larger than the middle third of the meniscus (Fig. 6.3). The pliable nature of the meniscus must not be forgotten. Hall (1978) has drawn attention to the 'buckled' meniscus during arthrography, which maybe misinterpreted as damaged.

7.4.5 Degenerative changes of the menisci

The radiologist cannot see degeneration on arthrography. He can only observe the changes of meniscal damage classically associated with histological evidence of degeneration. Degeneration may be present with and without a meniscal tear; the increasing tendency for the orthopaedic surgeon to retain menisci where possible means that the diagnosis of degeneration will not lead to meniscectomy unless pressing clinical considerations require it.

Degenerative change is characterized by minor irregularities or small surface tears of the menisci with surface absorption of positive contrast medium. Tears, particularly those with a horizontal element, may be associated with such changes.

It would be wrong to regard degeneration of the menisci (or, indeed, equivalent degeneration of the fibrocartilage of the intervertebral discs) as a spontaneous event unrelated to activity. The relative loss of elasticity with ageing is compounded by repeated episodes of minor trauma to structures which do not heal spontaneously.

The early stages of degenerative cleavage tears are not demonstrable arthrographically if, as Smillie says, they begin centrally in the relatively inelastic meniscus

(Smillie, 1970). Only when the tear extends to the surface (Fig. 3.3b) can it be revealed.

The relationship between degenerative joint disease and meniscal lesions is not clear-cut. Damage to the articular cartilage leading to osteoarthrosis can follow both the removal of a meniscus, usually with some degree of instability of the knee, and the direct pressure of a retained bucket-handle tear during repeated locking episodes. In the presence of osteoarthrosis of sufficient degree to produce reduction in the thickness of the articular cartilage, it is unusual for the menisci to be entirely normal and often post-traumatic surface irregularities are observed. With increasing damage to the articular cartilage, degenerate fragmented menisci are a common finding.

The incidence of horizontal tears of the menisci increases with the severity of degenerative joint disease (Noble and Hamblen, 1975). However, it seems unlikely to be a direct relationship, because the cleavage lesion is more common in males, whereas the reverse is true in the case of osteoarthrosis. Also, whilst cleavage lesions of all sorts are twice as common in the medial meniscus (Noble and Hamblen, 1975), in many series osteoarthrosis is rather more frequent in the lateral compartment (Wiley, 1968). None of these points exclude the relationship, but they do raise the possibility that a variety of types of cleavage lesions exist, perhaps with different aetiologies. Necropsy studies (Noble and Hamblen, 1975) suggest that the incidence of such lesions in the elderly (60 per cent) indicates that a significant proportion are either symptomless or symptoms are ascribed to another pathology, such as osteoarthrosis.

7.4.6   Other causes of diagnostic error in relation to the meniscus

Perhaps the most unhelpful variation in technique is to use too much positive-contrast medium. In common with others at the time, it was our practice to use 5 to 6 ml 60 per cent meglumine iothalamate solution. This pools in the recesses of the joint, obscures some of the features and excessive coating can lead to the erroneous diagnosis of tears of the menisci. I have experimented in the reduction of the amount of medium employed to as little as 1 ml, which I found unsatisfactory for adequate surface coating in the average knee. As a routine, therefore, an average of 3 ml is used.

Of the various technical errors or omissions that can be made by the beginner in knee arthrography, incomplete examination of the posterior horn is the commonest. The cause usually lies in an unjustifiable preoccupation with the anterior horn and leaving only one or two spot films for the posterior horn. In these circumstances, as indeed with similar exploits with the duodenal cap in Barium studies, the beginner must expect to expose more spot films than the expert. It is not an overstatement of the case to reiterate that examination of the posterior horn of the meniscus is not complete until the condyles of the femur almost overlap (Figs. 7.15 and 7.17).

7.4.7 Loose bodies and artefacts

During the examination the arthrographer should not move the knee vigorously or foaming will occur with the production of many bubbles. These produce curvilinear densities at their interfaces, which may suggest or obscure meniscal tears. When loose bodies are suspected clinically, the presence of bubbles is a great hindrance to diagnosis and, for this reason, single contrast gas arthrography is sometimes to be preferred when only this question needs to be answered.

Loose bodies and meniscal fragments may remain hidden in the intercondylar region of the femur, unless demonstrable by specific intercondylar views (Hall, 1978). We have little personal knowledge of the value of this technique, with no available angulation of the tubes on the fluoroscopic tables used for arthrography.

7.4.8 Calcification and ossification of the meniscus

Calcification in the articular cartilage indicates chondrocalcinosis, for which a variety of causes exist, the commonest probably being calcium pyrophosphate deposition disease (pseudogout) (Jensen and Putnam, 1975, Resnick *et al.*, 1977).

Calcification of the meniscus has been described in linear and punctate forms by McCarty *et al.* (1966), who believe that the linear variety is related to chondrocalcinosis. Schubert and Pras (1968) have shown that degeneration of the fibrocartilaginous intervertebral disc is accompanied by a loss of chondroitin sulphate and that this predisposes to the deposition of calcium phosphate.

As meniscal calcification is twice as common in menisci (of similar age) with cleavage tears (Noble and Hamblen, 1975), a similar mechanism to that operating in the intervertebral disc may exist. The identification of calcification in the soft tissues of the joint is one important reason for obtaining plain films prior to arthrography. Surface calcification is obscured by the introduction of positive-contrast medium and, even when calcification is present in the extrasynovial tissues or the depth of the meniscus, it may be difficult to establish with certainty that the density is not due to the medium.

Although constantly present in certain other mammals, the presence of ossicles in human menisci is rare. In 1942, Weaver found only ten reported cases; by 1972, Symeonides and Ionnides had managed to record a further eight cases, including three of their own. The patient, usually a young adult, presents with pain following trauma and a meniscal tear is suspected. Plain films show a radio-opaque body in the tibio-femoral space, which may be mistaken for a loose body within the synovial cavity. Aetiological views vary between such ossicles being vestigal and post-traumatic. The invariable unilateral involvement and the occasional report of development of ossification over a period of years following injury (Symeonides and Ionnides, 1972) makes the post-traumatic thesis more likely. They have been described in both medial and lateral menisci.

7.4.9 Problems of technique contributing to a suboptimal examination

The diagnostic accuracy is usually reduced when the examination is of poor technical quality. Table 7.6 details some of the causes for technical problems and their solution.

Table 7.6 Reasons for technical problems and their correction

Problem	Cause	Solution
Unable to inject gas	Needle not free in joint or blocked	(1) Try and inject small amount whilst withdrawing the needle (2) Change needle (for smaller size) (3) Try new site or other side of knee
Gas in joint, but no positive contrast	(1) Local anaesthetic (not contrast) injected (2) Contrast medium injected outside joint	(1) Check sterile tray (2) Screen for evidence of contrast medium in peri-articular tissues
Suprapatellar pouch does not distend with gas	(1) Needle outside joint (2) Needle in joint, synovial cavity ruptured or leaking	(1) Reposition needle (2) Do the best you can, if necessary single-contrast examination
Enough contrast and gas in joint, but gas does not separate condyles	(1) Band or patient has slipped (2) Screening wrong side of knee	Reposition
Poor detail	(1) Synovitis (2) Damaged cartilage (3) Delay in examination	(1) Make sure all effusion is aspirated (2) Diagnostic feature

7.5 Illustrative cases

This chapter ends with a number of arthrograms to illustrate certain problems and features. In order that the reader may test his diagnostic ability, the section has been arranged with the illustration and caption on the left hand page and the diagnostic description on the right, so that the latter may be covered up if so desired.

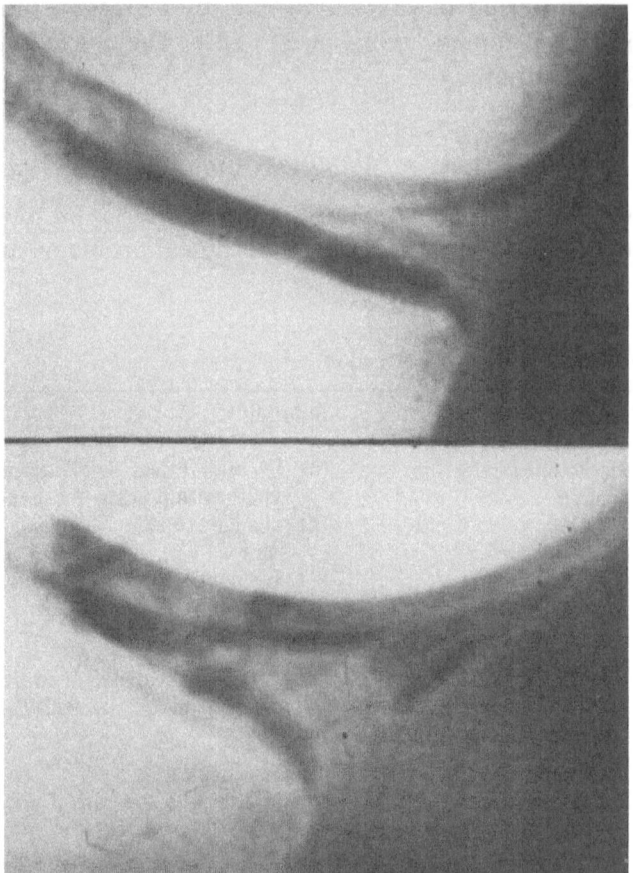

Fig. 7.1 A 45-year-old man who had had a medial
meniscetomy 6 years earlier for a bucket-handle tear.
18 months prior to the present attendance, he had
suffered a twisting injury to the knee, since when he
had experienced a number of locking episodes. Plain
X-ray normal. Clinical diagnosis: retained posterior
horn following meniscectomy.

Tear of posterior horn remnant.
A slightly large remnant of the posterior horn remains.
More anteriorly (upper film) a suggestion of a
horizontal tear is shown; posteriorly a small fragment
has been detached from the tip of the posterior horn
remnant and it is this that, no doubt, accounts for the
locking episodes. The tear of the posterior horn
remnant was confirmed at arthroscopy and arthrotomy.

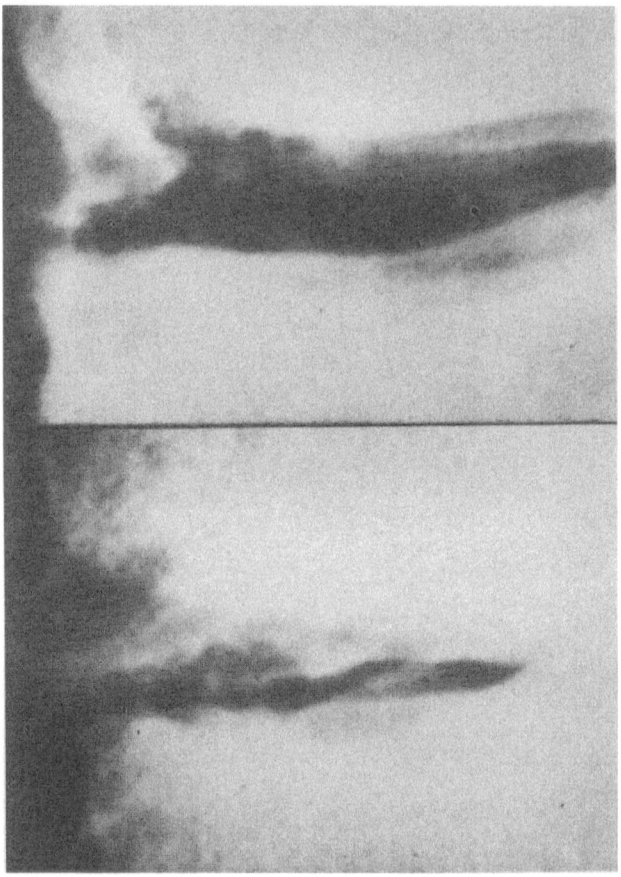

Fig. 7.2 A 37-year-old male patient who had had a lateral meniscectomy 17 years earlier and removal of loose bodies from the same knee 6 years ago. He complained of pain in the knee, but no locking. The clinical diagnosis was of a tear of the medial meniscus and/or a remnant of the lateral meniscus. Plain films showed degenerative change and possible loose bodies. The film shown here is of the posterior horn of the lateral meniscus.

Tear of posterior horn of meidal meniscus.
Arthroscopy in this case showed a normal anterior two-thirds of the meniscus with a suggestion of a split in the posterior horn; the lateral meniscus showed an abnormal posterior horn remnant. Arthrography confirmed the appearances of the lateral meniscus and showed that the posterior horn of the medial meniscus was grossly abnormal with a vertical tear of its substance. The articular cartilage over the tibial condyle is lost and some irregularity of that over the femoral condyle is present. The presence of such degenerative change probably contributes to the suboptimal clarity of the picture.

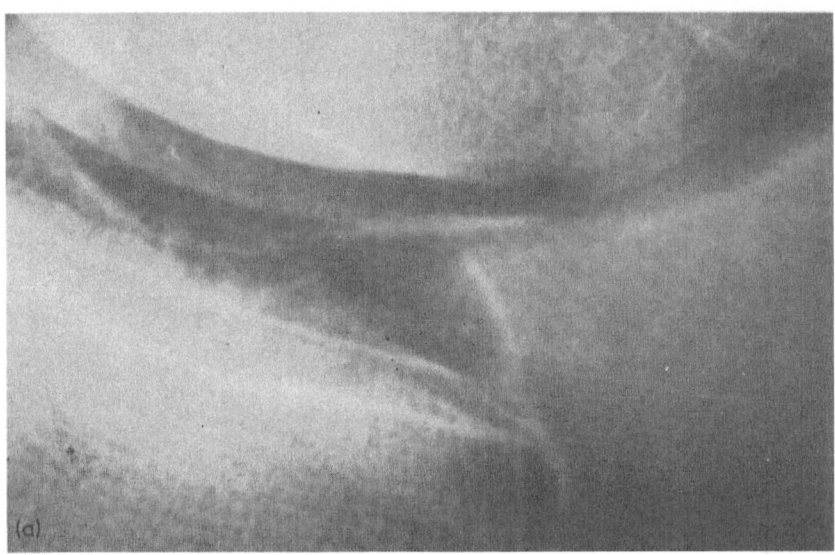

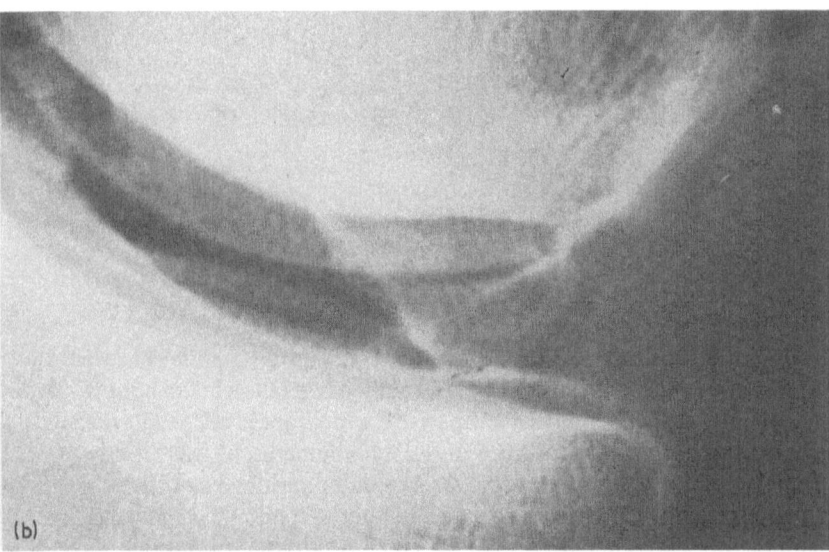

Fig. 7.3 A 33-year-old man whose knee had not been normal since a skiing injury 6 years earlier. Pain and clicking, but no locking episode. Clinical diagnosis:? injury of medial meniscus. Plain films normal. Arthrographic views of medial meniscus: (a) anterior, (b) middle, (c) posterior.

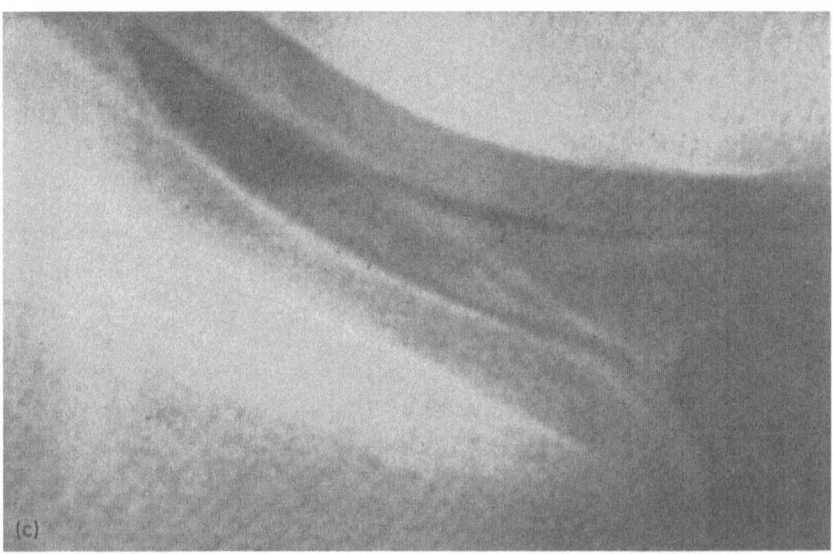

Bucket-handle tear of medial meniscus.
The anterior horn is short and shows an indistinct margin. In addition, a possible fragment is visible in the joint space. A vertical peripheral tear of the meniscus is shown on the other films, indicating that damage has been inflicted on the whole meniscus. The appearances suggest that the bucket-handle has become detached anteriorly. The findings were confirmed at operation.

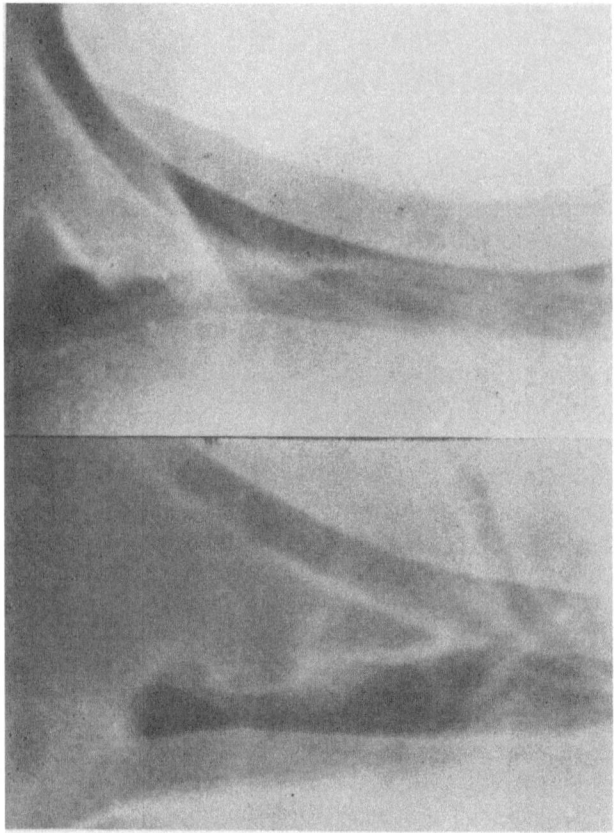

Fig. 7.4 A 42-year-old man who injured his knee
jumping off a trailer 4 years earlier. Since then he had
experienced pain, giving way, but no true locking. Plain
films were normal. Clinical diagnosis: ? torn meniscus,
side not apparent. Films illustrated are of the medial
meniscus.

Detached bucket-handle tear of medial meniscus.
The tear was not demonstrated at arthrography. A
comment was made that the meniscal surface appeared
irregular, suggesting degeneration. The lower film of
the posterior horn shows what appears to be a partial
tear of its under-surface and it is possible that this
extended to become a complete detachment in the
2 months between arthrography and operation.
Conclusion: arthrographic error, failure to demonstrate
tear.

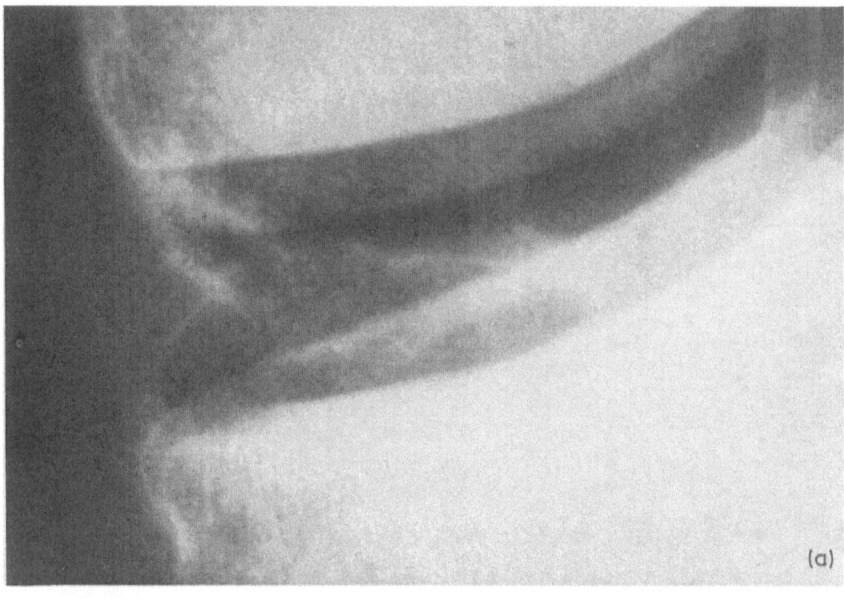

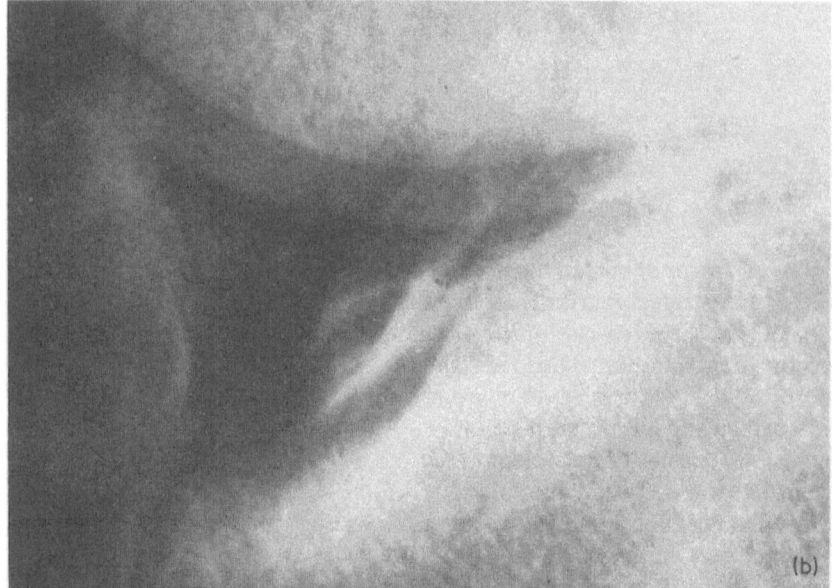

Fig. 7.5 A 22-year-old man who experienced a twisting injury of his knee 6 years earlier. Locking occurred for the first time a year before this presentation and since then he had suffered a further significant injury to the knee at squash. No specific clinical diagnosis was made and plain films showed early degenerative change in all compartments of the knee. The films show the anterior and posterior horns of the lateral meniscus.

Extensive tear of lateral meniscus.
(a) A short peripheral remnant of the anterior horn is present with the detached fragment lying on the surface of the tibial condyle. (b) The detachment of the posterior horn is evident. The patient received no immediate treatment as he remained completely free from all symptoms for 1 year after the arthrogram! The arthrographic findings were confirmed at arthroscopy and operation some 14 months after arthrography.

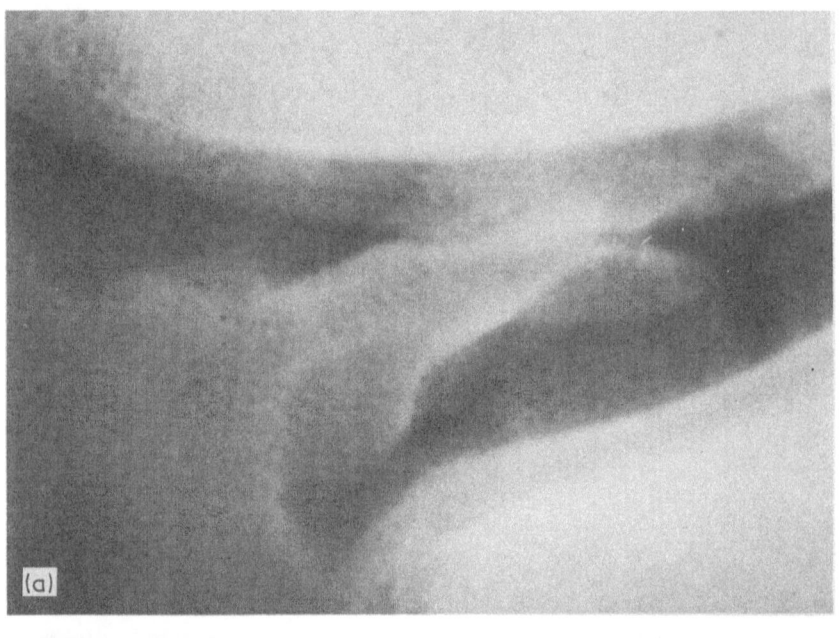

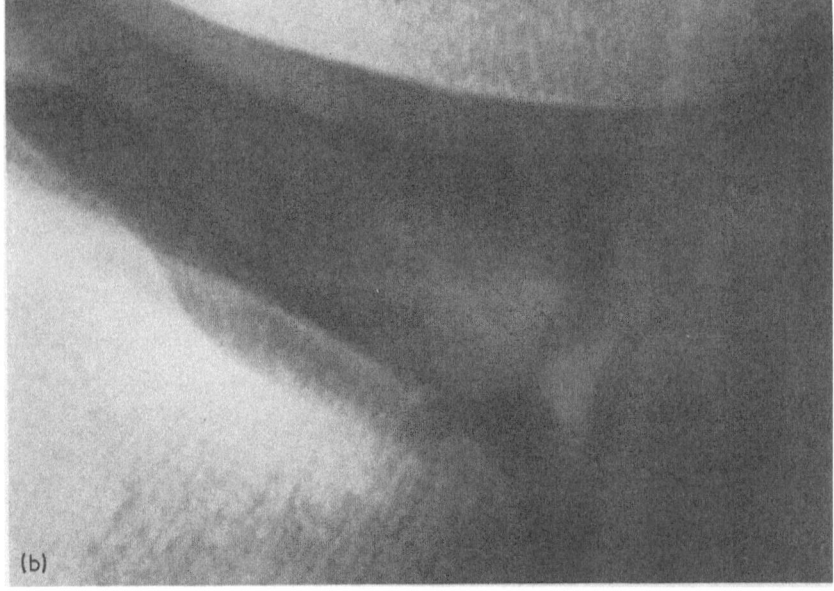

Fig. 7.6 A 32-year-old man who complained of recurrent pain in his knee in the year following an injury. Plain films showed only minimal evidence of degenerative change. The clinical diagnosis was ? torn lateral meniscus. (a) Anterior horn medial meniscus (b) posterior horn lateral meniscus.

Tear of lateral meniscus.
The shape of the anterior horn of the medial meniscus was commented on by the
arthrographer, who queried the possibility of a small horizontal tear. The major lesion
lay in the lateral meniscus, however, which showed a large peripheral tear of its
posterior horn. This was described at operation as a parrot-beak tear. The medial
meniscus was not inspected as no symptoms or signs were related to that side of the
knee. Conclusion: arthrographic diagnosis of lateral meniscus tear confirmed,
although the nature of the tear was not agreed.

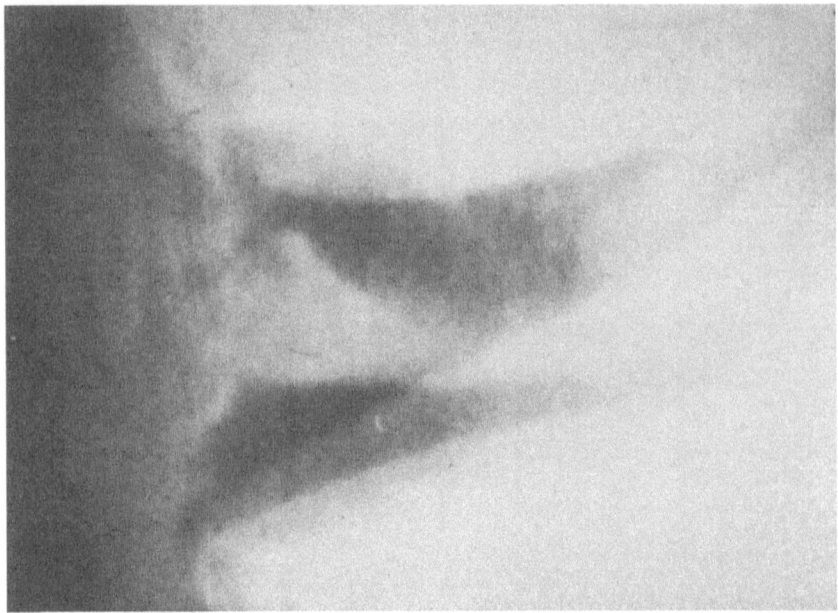

Fig. 7.7 A 26-year-old man with a history of injury 6 months previously. The knee gave a periodic painful click located on the lateral side of the joint. A tear of the lateral meniscus was diagnosed clinically. Plain X-rays were normal, apart from slight widening of the lateral joint space, suggesting a discoid meniscus. Films of anterior horn of lateral meniscus.

Detachment of discoid lateral meniscus.
The film shows a peripheral detachment of the anterior horn with absorption of contrast medium into the surface of the meniscus. Despite a suspect plain film, the arthrographer was not prepared to call the meniscus discoid, although this was the surgeon's opinion. The tear extended into the posterior horn, which was only partially detached.

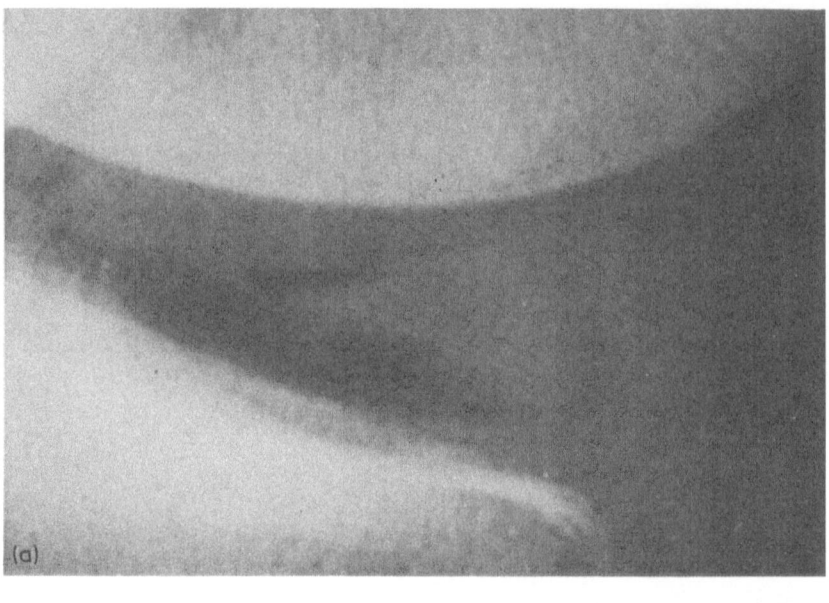

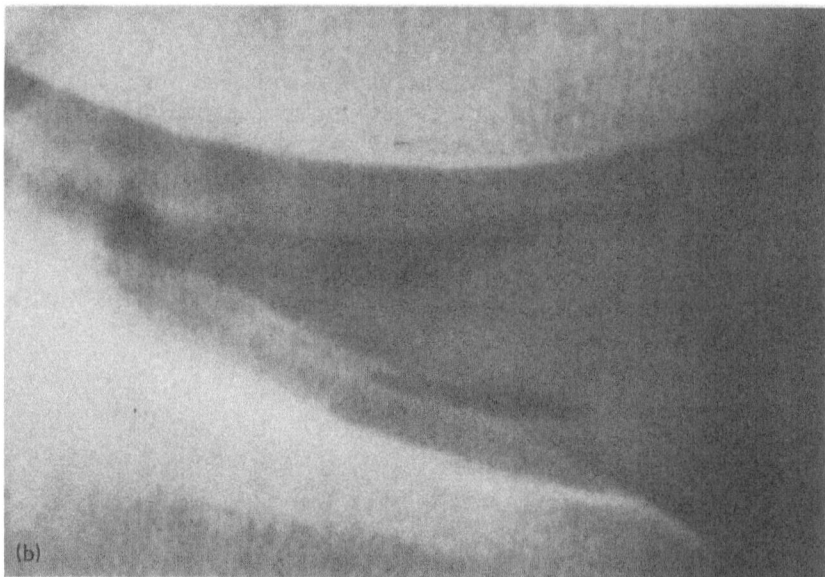

Fig. 7.8 A 36-year-old man with a 4-year history of pain in the knee. No firm clinical diagnosis; normal plain films. Two views of the medial meniscus are provided, (a) and (b).

Tear of medial meniscus.
Poor coating has been obtained, perhaps as a result of the associated synovitis. The meniscus shows an irregular free edge with absorption of medium into its substance, a feature which led the radiologist to diagnose a torn degenerate meniscus. The surgeon interpreted the appearance as a parrot-beak tear, but his line drawing exactly simulated the radiologist's description. Conclusion: Full correlation of findings; terminological divergence of opinion.

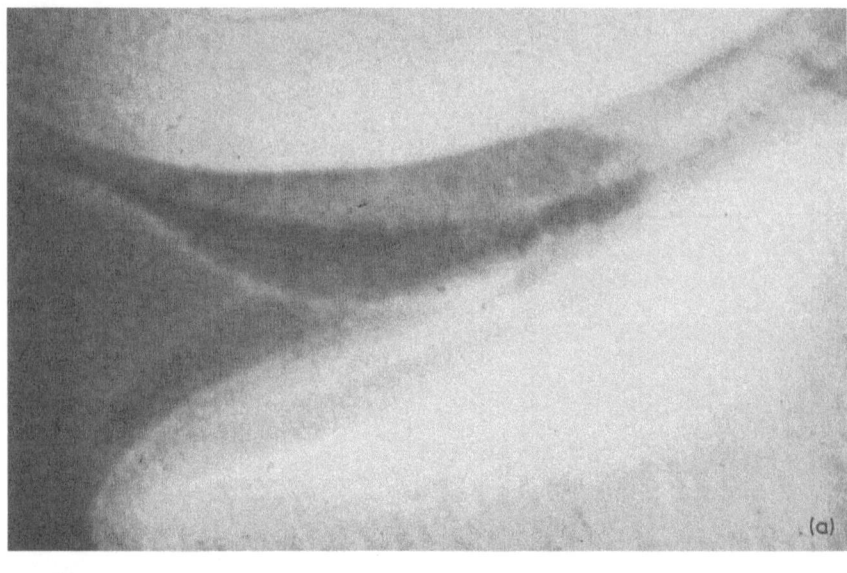

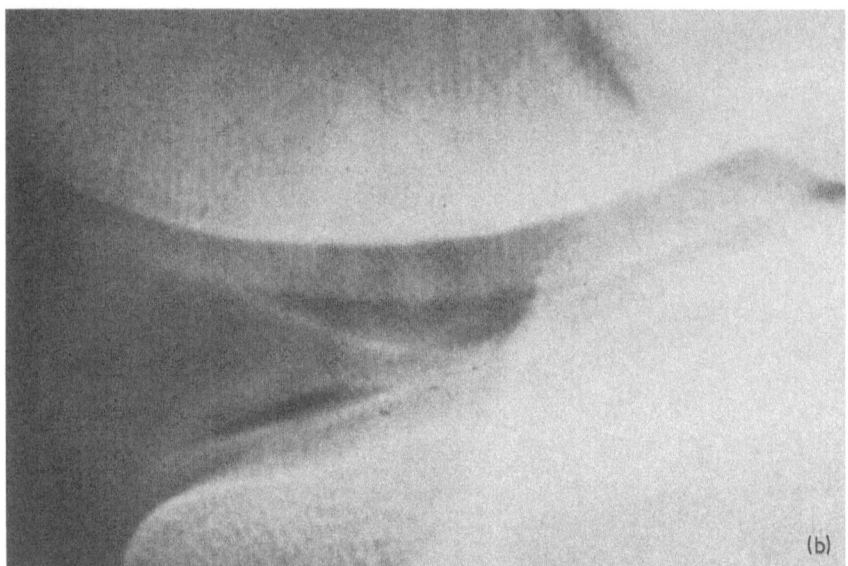

Fig. 7.9 A 33-year-old woman with a 6-year history of retropatellar pain. Her history and signs were consistent with a diagnosis of chondromalacia patellae but, in addition, she exhibited a positive McMurray test, suggesting a coincidental meniscal lesion. Plain films were normal. The films shown are two views, (a) and (b), of the lateral meniscus.

Parrot-beak tear of partially discoid meniscus.
The arthrogram was reported as normal. Rescrutiny reveals the meniscus to be abnormally short in its anterior half (a). The posterior horn (b) shows an indistinct free margin due to an overlying flap of the adjoining edge. This should not have been assessed as normal and more views should have been obtained to elucidate the anatomy. Arthroscopy, confirmed by arthrotomy, revealed a slightly discoid meniscus with a small parrot-beak tear of its margin. Conclusion: arthrographic error of interpretation.

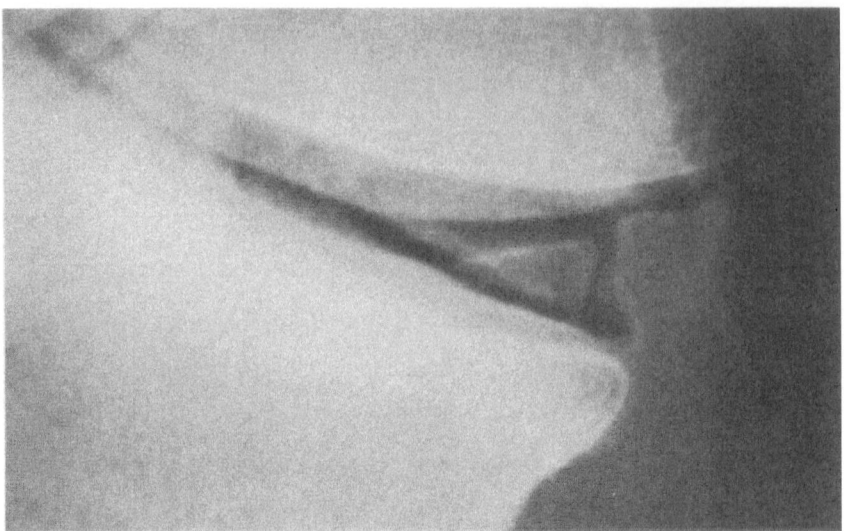

Fig. 7.10 A 25-year-old man with a 7-month history of pain in the knee. 2 years before, the patient had had a lateral meniscectomy for a bucket-handle tear; this operation had been preceded by arthroscopy and, at that time, the medial meniscus was reported as normal. The current clinical diagnosis rested between a tear of the medial meniscus and a residual remnant of the lateral meniscus now causing symptoms. Plain films were normal. The medial meniscus is illustrated.

Bucket-handle tear of the medial meniscus.
A classical vertical tear is shown, consistent with the diagnosis of a bucket-handle tear. This was confirmed at operation.

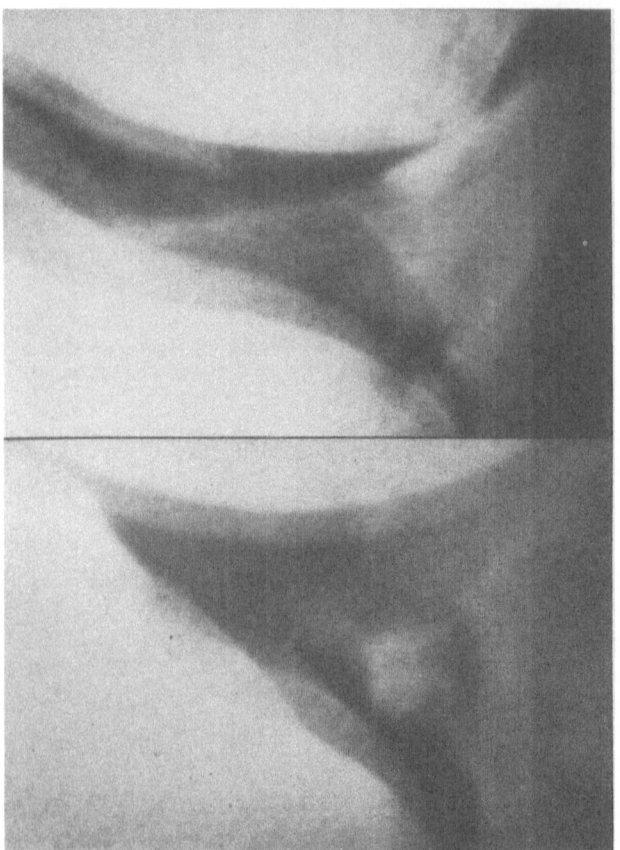

Fig. 7.11 A 22-year-old man with a history of
rotational injury to his knee. Plain films were normal
and the clinical diagnosis varied between one of a tear
of the lateral meniscus to 'meniscal injury? side'
depending on the signs at successive clinic attendances.
The lateral meniscus is illustrated.

Extensive tear of lateral meniscus with detached posterior horn.
The medial meniscus was normal. The films show an irregular short peripheral remnant of the meniscus; the detached rim or meniscus cannot be visualized.
Operation confirmed the arthrographic findings but, in addition, revealed the displaced fragment of the bucket-handle tear in the intercondylar region of the knee.

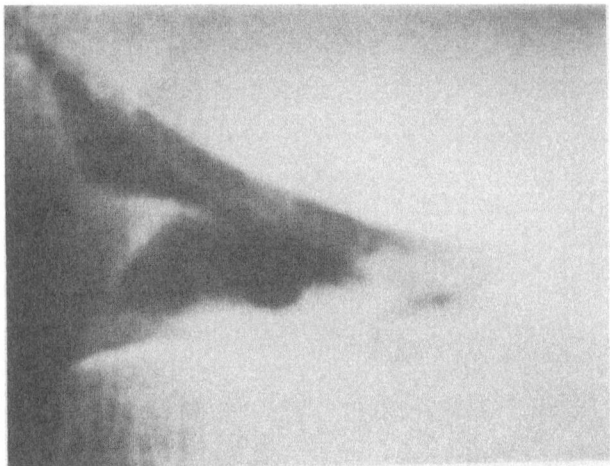

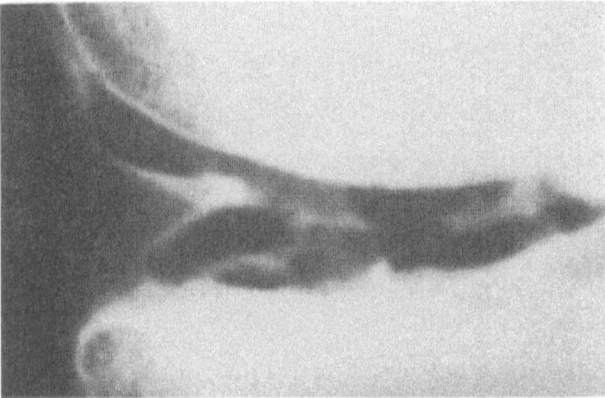

Fig. 7.12 A 31-year-old woman whose only injury was being struck on the knee 16 years before by a hockey ball. She had had trouble on and off, but 2 months ago the knee gave way. Plain films normal: Clinical diagnosis: chondromalacia patellae or torn medial meniscus.

Tear of medial meniscus (old).
The medial meniscus is small, indicating that loss of its
substance has occurred. The presence of fragments on
the tibial plateau should be observed. Although the
films are not ideal (this was an early case in the series)
the arthrographer was able to suggest that regeneration
and repair following an old tear best explained the
findings. At arthroscopy and operation, a torn tag of
the meniscus was found to be attached posteriorly. Loss
of articular cartilage, shown on the tibial surface of the
lower arthrographic film, was also observed at
arthroscopy.

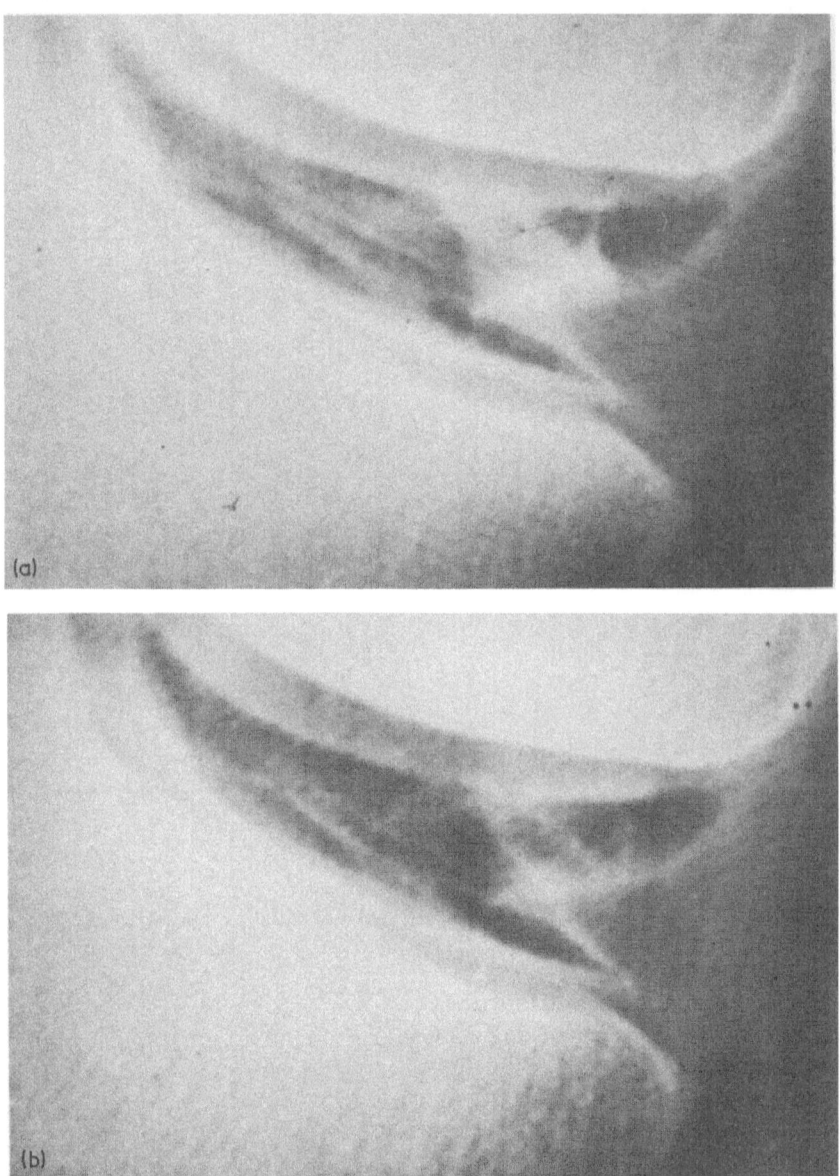

Fig. 7.13 A 42-year-old man complained of pain and locking of his knee. Plain films were normal and a clinical diagnosis of a medial meniscus tear was made. The films are of the medial meniscus.

Tear of medial meniscus.
In both views (a) and (b) the meniscus is short and irregular with absorption of medium into its damaged edge. The radiologist called this a bucket-handle tear, but it clearly is more complex than that. At operation, the surgeon designated the injury a parrot-beak tear.

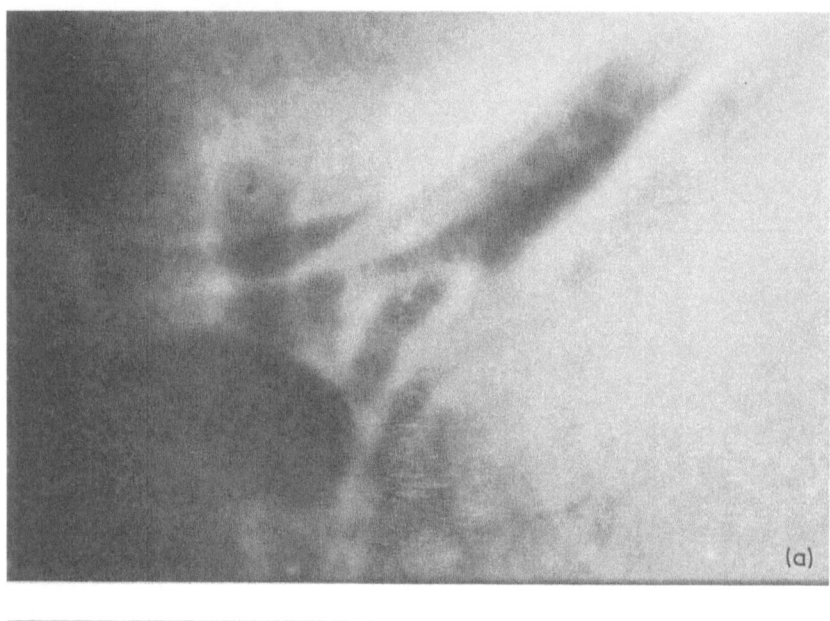

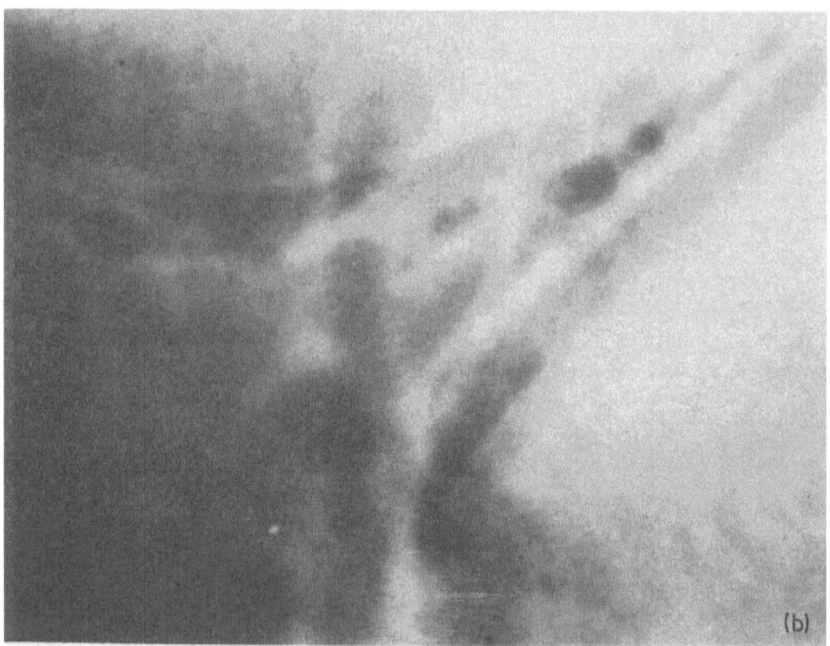

Fig. 7.14 A 45-year-old man with 6-month history of giving way of knee. Medial meniscectomy had been performed 18 months earlier. Plain films were normal. Clinical diagnosis: ? remnant remaining after medial meniscectomy +? anterior cruciate injury. Films, (a) and (b), are of the lateral meniscus.

Tear of lateral meniscus.
The lateral meniscus shows a small posterior horn which contains a horizontal tear.
The medial compartment (not illustrated) contained a normal post-meniscectomy
remnant. At operation, a bucket-handle tear of the lateral meniscus was
demonstrated. The detached fragment is not shown arthrographically.

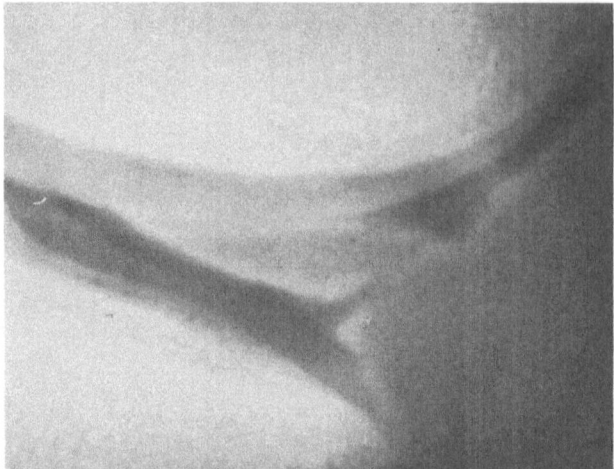

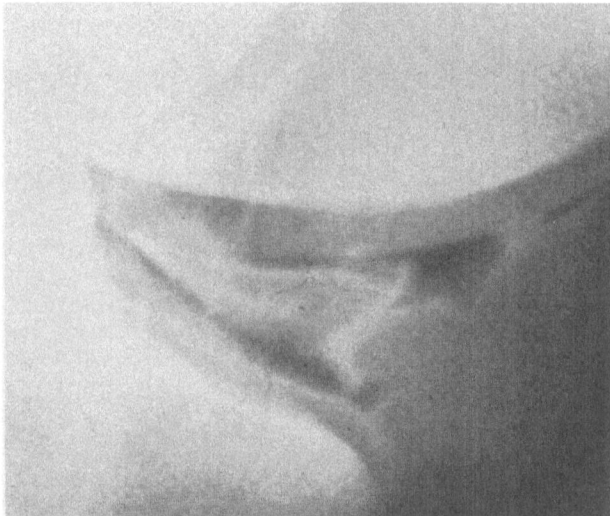

Fig. 7.15 A 19-year-old man who injured his knee
2 months earlier when landing after heading the ball at
football. Main complaints: swelling of the knee when
running, doubtful history of locking. Plain films show
a possible old osteochondral detachment from medial
femoral condyle. Films show medial meniscus.

Bucket-handle tear of medial meniscus.
The two films show complete tears of the peripheral
third of the medial meniscus, indicating a
bucket-handle tear of its posterior half. Operation
revealed some irregularity of the anterior horn of the
medial meniscus and meniscectomy was performed
without confirming the presence of a tear of the
posterior horn. Conclusion: Error by operating
surgeon. The posterior horn was probably removed
through the line of the tear.

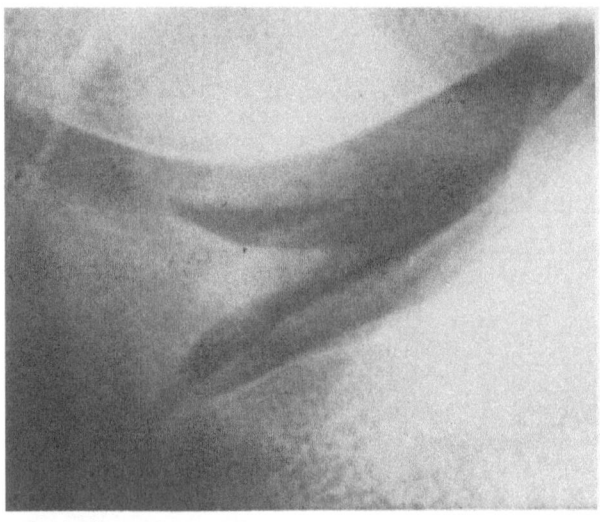

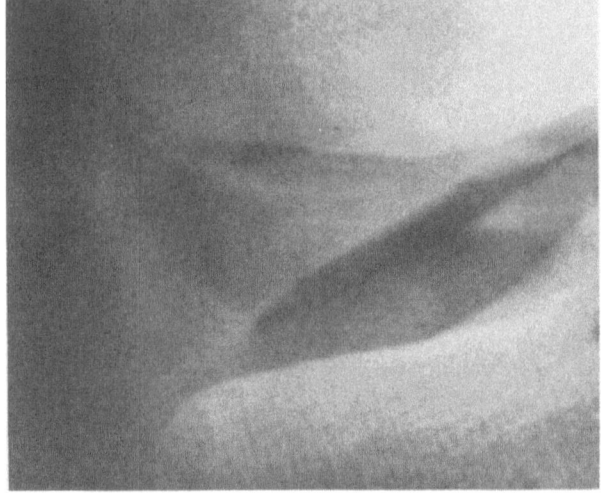

Fig. 7.16 A 21-year-old man with a troublesome knee for 1 year; a vague history of injury at football was obtained. Plain films were normal and a clinical diagnosis of a cystic lateral meniscus was made. A positive McMurray test was obtained in both knees and arthrography was requested. The illustration shows the lateral meniscus.

Parrot-beak tear of discoid lateral meniscus.
The arthrogram was reported to be normal; later
examination of the films showed this not to be the case.
Arthrographically, the meniscus did not appear to be
discoid. In the upper film, an abnormal meniscal
fragment overlies the meniscus shown in profile; this
cannot be explained on normal appearances and
indicates a flap-like tear of the free edge (parrot-beak
tear) involving the middle third. The posterior horn is
normal. Operation revealed a discoid meniscus with an
oblique parrot-beak tear of the free edge of the middle
third of the lateral meniscus. Conclusion: arthrographic
error – error of interpretation.

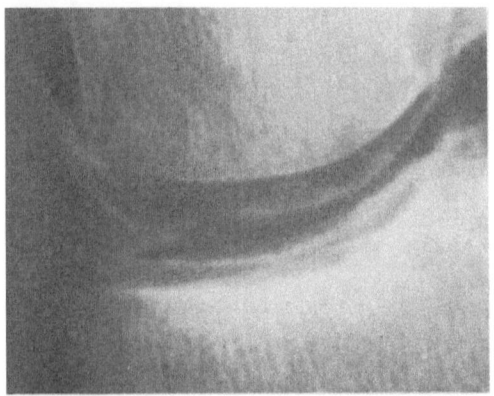

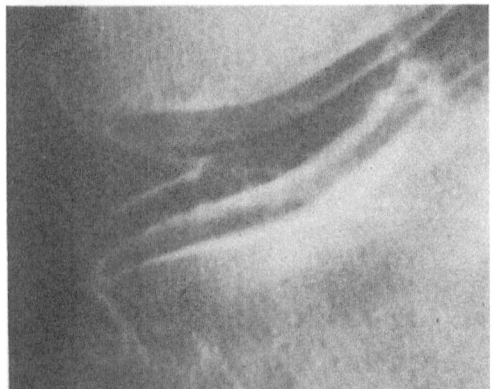

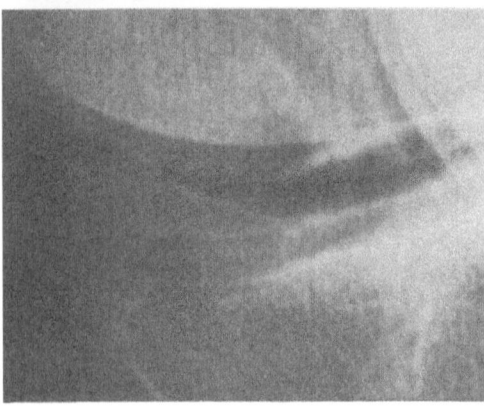

Fig. 7.17 A 51-year-old woman with persistent discomfort in the knee since a fall 2 years earlier. In addition, she experienced some more severe anteromedial pain, swelling, and had been unable to extend the knee fully. The plain X-ray examination revealed no abnormality, except for new bone formation in the intercondylar region, possibly associated with an anterior cruciate injury. Clinical diagnosis: tear of medial meniscus. Illustrated are arthrographic views of anterior half of medial meniscus.

Tear of anterior horn of medial meniscus.
The arthrogram was reported as showing no
tear, although the posterior horn of the
meniscus was described as showing early
degeneration. At operation the anterior
horn was torn, the posterior horn showed
fibrillation. Full extension of the knee was
achieved by 6 months following
meniscectomy. Conclusion: Arthrographic
error. Review of the arthrographic
appearances still does not provide evidence
of a significant abnormality of the anterior
horn.

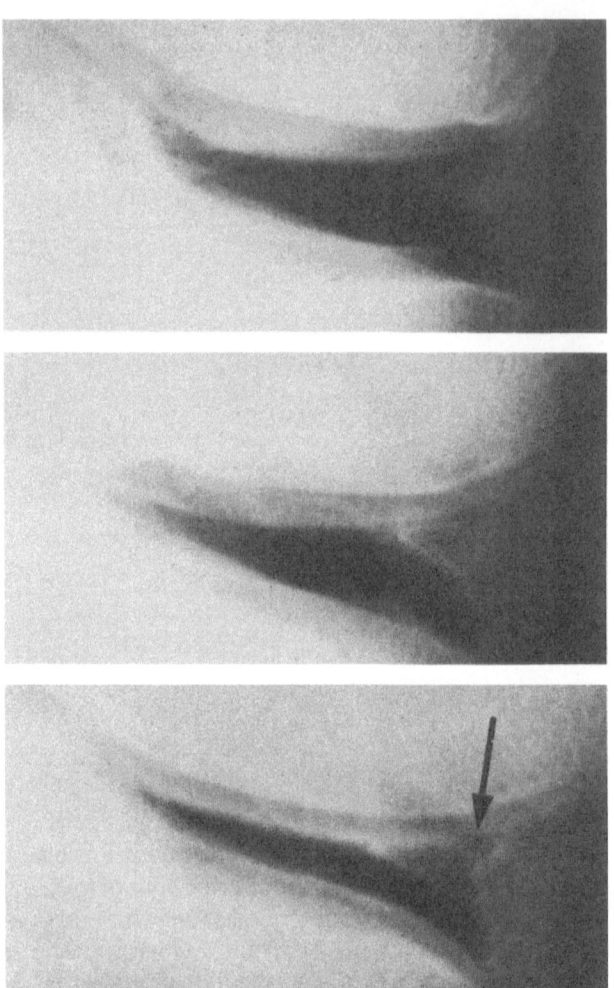

Fig. 7.18 A 29-year-old man with a 22-month history of
pain in the knee, localized to the medial side; no
locking. Plain films normal. Clinical diagnosis: minor
tear of medial meniscus. Films shown are of the medial
meniscus.

Bucket-handle tear of medial meniscus.
All the views shown reveal an abnormal medial
meniscus; anteriorly the meniscus is small with a
blunted margin and perhaps some absorption of
medium into its free edge. A vertical tear of the
posterior horn is demonstrated (arrow). This was one
of the earliest arthrograms performed at this Hospital.
Although this fact is reflected in the indifferent quality
of the examination, it also shows that a diagnostic
examination can be expected soon after the institution
of the investigation.

References

Brown, D.W., Allman, F.L. Jr. and Eaton, S.B. (1978). Knee arthrography, a comparison of radiographic and surgical findings in 295 cases. *American Journal of Sports Medicine,* **6**, 165–172.

Butt, W.P. and McIntyre, J.L. (1969). Double contrast arthrography of the knee. *Radiology,* **92**, 487–99.

Dalinka, M.K., Corren, G.S. and Wershba, M. (1973). Knee arthrography. *CRC Critical Reviews in Clinical Radiology and Nuclear Medicine,* **4**, 1–59.

Freiberger, R.H., Killoran, P.J. and Cardona, G. (1966).Arthrography of the knee by double contrast method. *American Journal of Roentgenology,* **97**, 736–47.

Hall, F.M. (1976). Pitfalls in knee arthrography. *Radiology,* **118**, 55–62.

Hall, F.M. (1978). Buckled meniscus. *Radiology,* **126**, 89–90.

Jackson, R.W. and Abe, I. (1972). The role of arthroscopy in the management of disorders of the knee. *Journal of Bone and Joint Surgery,* **54–B**, 310–22.

Jensen, P.S. and Putnam, C.E. (1975). Current concepts with respect to chondrocalcinosis and the pseudogout syndrome. *American Journal of Roentgenology,* **123**, 531–9.

Kiss, J. and Moir, J.D. (1968). Experience with arthrographic examination of the knee joint. *Journal of the Canadian Association of Radiologists,* **19**, 187–91.

McCarty, D.J. Jr, Hogan, J.M., Gatter, R.A. and Grossman, M. (1966). Studies on pathological calcification in human cartilage 1: Prevalence and types of crystal deposits in the menisci of 215 cadavers. *Journal of Bone and Joint Surgery,* **48–A**, 309–25.

Noble, J. and Hamblen, D.L. (1975). The pathology of the degenerate meniscus lesion. *Journal of Bone and Joint Surgery,* **57–B**, 180–6.

Resnick, D., Niwayama, G., Goergen, T.G., Utsinger, P.D., Shapiro, R.F., Haselwood, D.H. and Wiesner, K.B. (1977). Clinical, radiographic and pathologic abnormalities in calcium pyrophosphate dihydrate deposition disease (CPPD). Pseudogout. *Radiology,* **122**, 1–15.

Ricklin, P., Rüttimann, A. and Del Buono, M.S. (1971). *Meniscus Lesions.* Georg Thieme Verlag, Stuttgart.

Schubert, M., Pras, M. (1968). Ground substance protein polysaccharides and the precipitation of calcium phosphate. *Clinical Orthopedics,* **60**, 235–55.

Smillie, I.S. (1970). *Injuries of the Knee Joint,* 4th Edn. Livingstone, Edinburgh.

Symeonides, P.P. and Ionnides, G. (1972). Ossicles in the knee menisci. *Journal of Bone and Joint Surgery,* **54–A**, 1288–92.

Thijn, C.J.P. (1979). *Arthrography of the Knee Joint,* p. 59. Springer Verlag, Berlin, Heidelberg, New York.

Weaver, J.B. (1942). Calcification and ossification of the menisci. *Journal of Bone and Joint Surgery,* **24**, 873–82.

Wiley, A.M. (1968). Pathological and clinical aspects of degenerative disease of the knee. *Canadian Journal of Surgery,* **11**, 14–22.

8 Chondral and osteochondral lesions

8.1 Acute lesions of cartilage and bone

During arthrographic examination only a small proportion of the total area of articular cartilage is demonstrable. However, surface damage to the articular cartilage can often be demonstrated, although usually such lesions are found to be very much more extensive at arthroscopy or arthrotomy than was suspected by the radiologist.

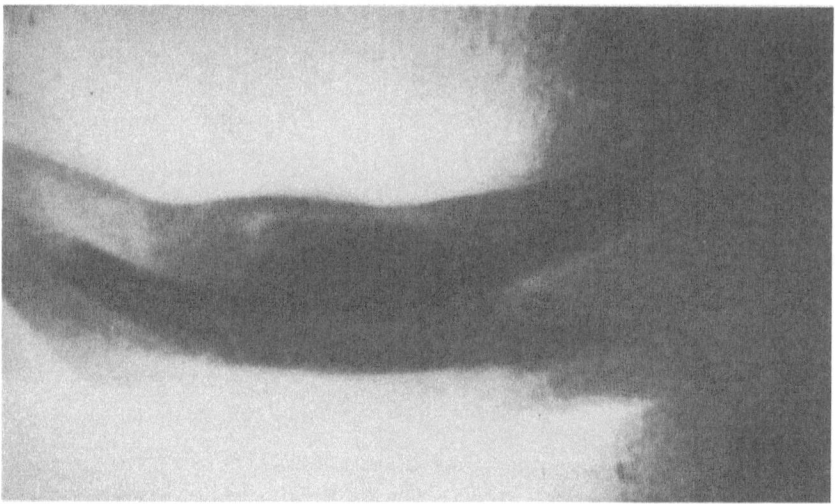

Fig. 8.1 *Traumatic erosion of articular cartilage.* A 26-year-old professional footballer developed a recurrent joint effusion in training. A medial meniscus lesion was suspected. Arthrography demonstrated that both menisci were intact, but that a defect of the articular cartilage of the medial femoral condyle was present. Arthrotomy subsequently confirmed these findings; the articular cartilage was deficient over an area of 3 cm×2 cm. A smaller area of articular cartilage loss was demonstrated over the lateral femoral condyle; this had not been shown at arthrography.

Damage to the articular cartilage and the underlying bone can result from blows tangential to its surface. It is likely that such injuries are common and that often the cartilage regenerates completely. More severe injuries and pressure damage from displaced menisci or joint incongruity secondary to ligament damage and instability lead to larger erosions (Fig. 8.1). These show as well-defined depressions of the articular margin.

Damage to the menisci is common when severe osteochondral fractures of the tibial plateau are sustained (Figs. 8.2, 8.3). Arthrography has also been used in the

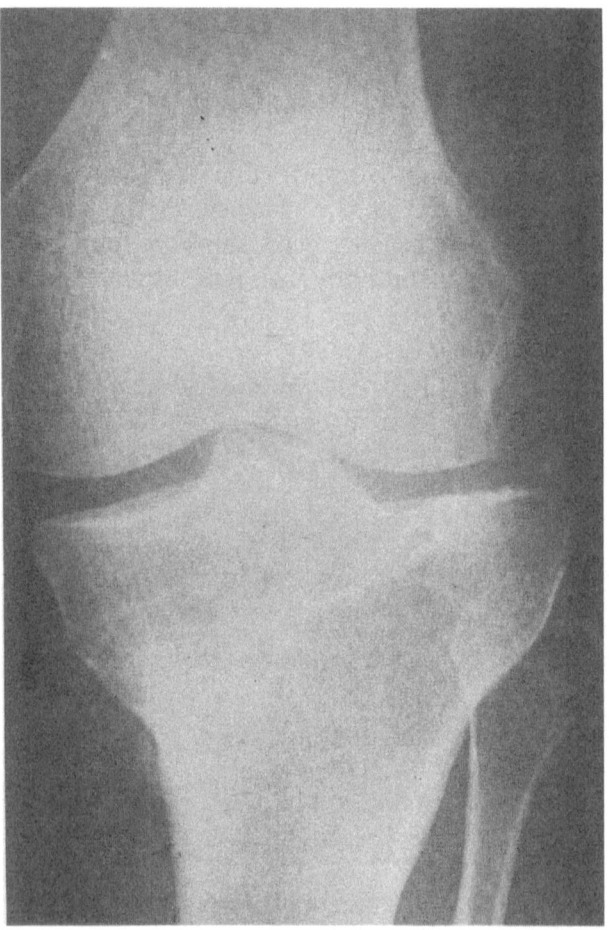

Fig. 8.2 *Meniscal damage associated with fracture of the tibial plateau.* The plain film shows a healed fracture of the proximal tibia, which has extended to involve the lateral articular surface.

evaluation of fractures of the tibial plateau (Anderson *et al.*, 1976), arthrotomography in articular lesions, particularly of the post-meniscectomy knee (Anderson and

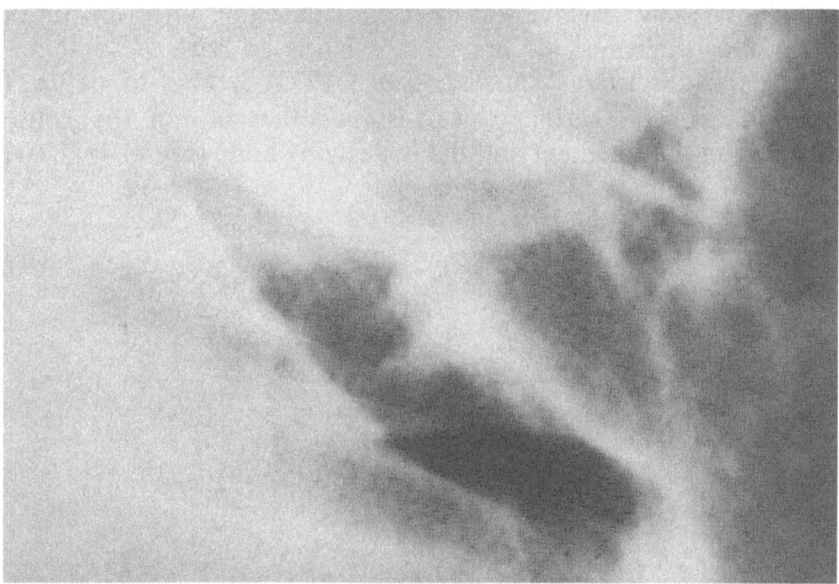

Fig. 8.3 The arthrogram demonstrates the damaged posterior horn of the lateral meniscus, which has lost its normal triangular shape and shows absorption of contrast medium into its surface. The patient, a 21-year-old woman, had had a lateral meniscectomy 1 year earlier; the appearances were correctly interpreted as a retained posterior horn. Considerable damage to the articular cartilage covering the lateral tibial condyle was revealed at arthrotomy.

Maslin, 1974), osteochondral fractures of the patella (Ashby *et al.*, 1975) and in penetrating injuries of the knee (Fordham and Turner, 1976). None of these is a common indication, but show that arthrography can be helpful in selected injuries.

8.2 The post-traumatic dissecans lesion

Post-traumatic osteochondral dissecting lesions of the knee, so-called osteochondritis dissecans, are found not uncommonly between the ages of 10 and 20 years, predominantly (4:1) in males (Aichroth, 1971). The site most often involved is the convex lateral aspect of the medial femoral condyle anteriorly. Concave articular surfaces are almost never affected. The findings and the treatment depend upon the extent and stage of the disorder. When the osteochondral fragment separates completely, it becomes a loose body, which may reattach to the synovium out of harm's way in the posterior compartment or the intercondylar region; some fragments may even be resorbed. In this instance a defect is left in the femoral condyle, which is usually identified easily on the plain radiograph, particularly the intercondylar projection. If, however, the fragment remains *in situ*, the plain film cannot demonstrate whether the overlying articular cartilage is intact or not, and therefore whether the osteochondral fragment is likely to heal.

Arthrography in this disorder (Wershba *et al.*, 1975) is able to define the overlying surface of articular cartilage, showing whether or not the contrast medium passes between the fragment and the underlying bone (Fig. 8.4). Usually

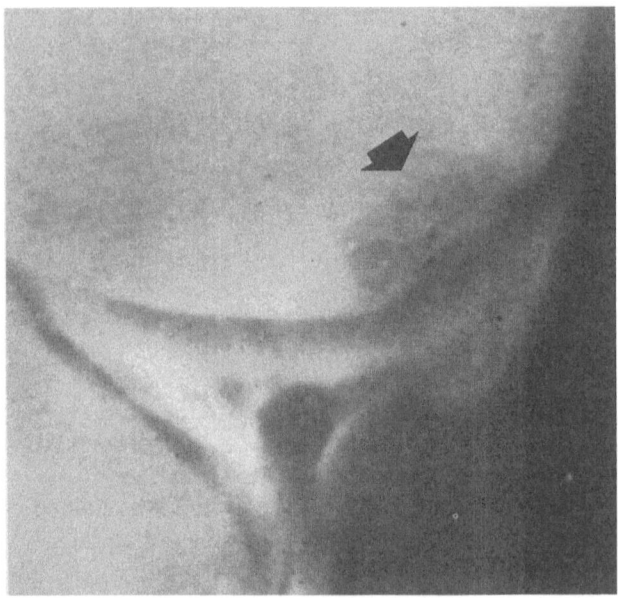

Fig. 8.4 *Osteochondral defect* of the posterior aspect of the lateral femoral condyle (arrow) shown at arthrography in an adolescent girl suspected of having a lateral meniscal tear; no tear of either meniscus was demonstrated. The patient's symptoms developed during a period of competitive swimming, employing mainly the breast stroke.

the articular cartilage is intact, indicating that healing is possible and only rarely is dissection complete (Nicholas *et al.*, 1970). Such information may influence future surgical management. Loose bodies and unsuspected lesions of the menisci may be revealed. At a later stage the condylar defect, from which an osteochondral fragment has dissected, may fill with fibrocartilage and this healing process can also be shown by arthrography.

8.3 Loose bodies

These may arise from dissecans lesions, other osteochondral trauma, degenerative joint disease, synovial osteochondromatosis (see p. 160), synovial fragments

(Staple, 1972), etc. A plain film is essential to locate any opaque elements in the loose bodies present. Very frequently, apparently loose particles are no longer free in the joint, but have gained attachment to a synovial surface.

Positive-contrast arthrography is of little value in the demonstration of loose bodies; either gas arthrography or a double-contrast technique, preferably employing a small amount (1 to 2 ml) of positive-contrast medium, is needed. An associated effusion is to be expected and must be aspirated prior to arthrography. Not only is the objective to confirm the presence of a loose body (Fig. 8.5 a,b),

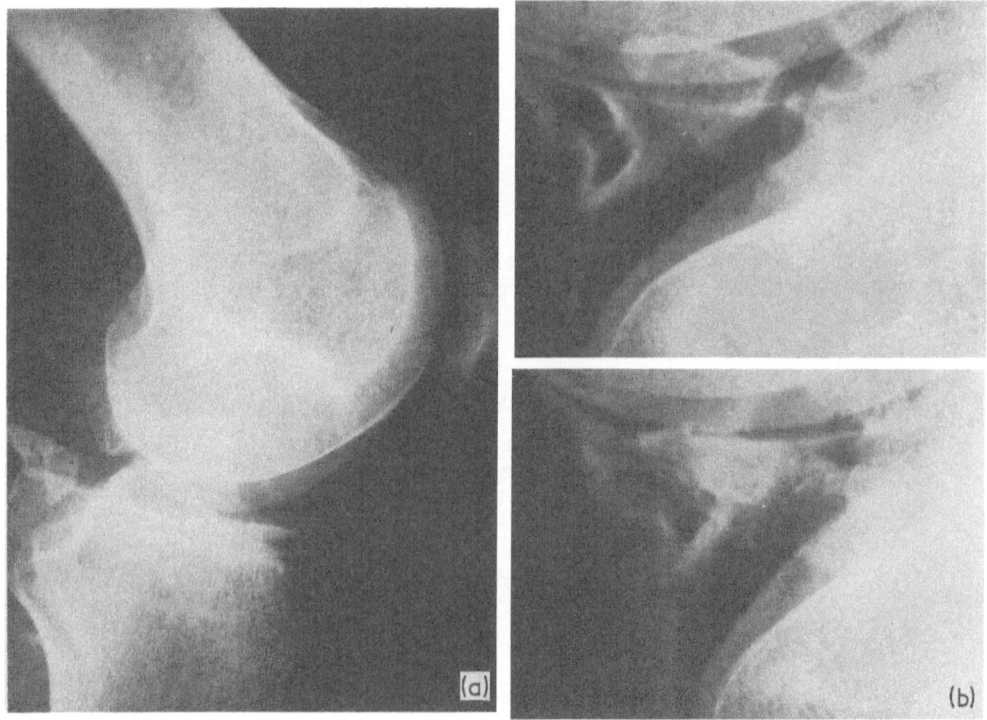

Fig. 8.5 *Loose bodies in knee.* A 35-year-old man presented with continuing pain in his knee for 10 years after a motor accident. (a) The plain lateral film shows irregularly shaped loose bodies in the posterior compartment. (b) Arthrography revealed no meniscal damage, but loose bodies overlie the posterior horn of the lateral meniscus.

taking special care to examine the recesses and bursae of the joint but, if possible, its site of origin should be determined by examination of all articular surfaces for osteochondral defects.

8.4 Chondromalacia patellae

Arthrography has little, if any, place in the management of this disorder. The early diagnosis is clinical and no arthrographic feature is present.

At a later stage, absorption of contrast medium and erosion of cartilage (Fig. 8.6)

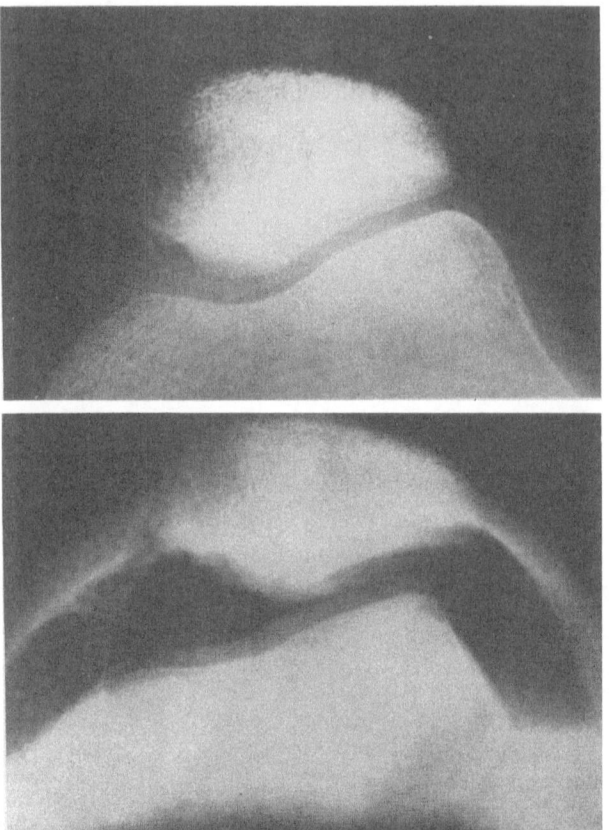

Fig. 8.6 *Post-traumatic loss of patellar articular cartilage*. This 14-year-old girl was a keen ballet performer. She complained increasingly of pain in her knee. The axial view of the patella shows irregularity of the subchondral bone of the medial articular facet. The axial view during arthrography shows loss of and irregularity of the articular cartilage overlying the abnormal bone. These appearances indicate a relatively late stage of chondromalacia patellae.

may be observed arthrographically. If, at this stage, the clinical findings are not clear (Staple, 1972) it seems likely that some other cause for symptoms exists. Arthroscopy has more to offer in the diagnosis of lesions of the articular cartilage than arthrography, though even with this technique the clinical significance of minor fibrillatory surface change is doubtful.

Although perhaps the majority of arthrographers (Nicholas *et al.*,1970, Dalinka *et al.*, 1973) share the view expressed here that the management of chondromalacia patellae is clinical and that the accuracy of arthrography in this disorder is insufficient to make it a worthwhile diagnostic method, other authors take an opposing view. Horns (1977) recommends the employment of a double-contrast technique and claims an accuracy, in arthrographic diagnosis of rupture confirmed at operation, of 87.5 per cent in a small series of 24 patients over a period of 2 years. The problem of the false positive diagnosis, so disturbing to other arthrographers, is not mentioned in this paper.

Thijn (1979) has written of his extensive experience and expertise in the diagnosis of patellar chondropathy. He describes a technique for careful examination of the articular cartilage but, even with his experience, a 29 per cent incidence of false negative and a 17 per cent of false positive results are found.

Whilst I believe the patellar articular cartilage should always be examined, when relevant, during arthrography, this examination is vastly inferior to arthroscopy and should not be performed as an elective procedure to establish such a diagnosis. As the establishment of the diagnosis of chondromalacia patellae rarely leads to specific therapy, a clinical diagnosis of the disorder is usually sufficient. When more accurate assessment is required, arthroscopy is the examination of choice and can grade the degree of chondropathy, if so desired (Thijn, 1979).

8.5 Complications of fractures of the tibial plateau

Anderson *et al.* (1976) have used arthrotomography in the evaluation of patients with problems following such fractures. This has provided good delineation of the articular surfaces. Useful information obtained includes the presence of torn or degenerate menisci (Figs. 8.2, 8.3), non-union of bone fragments, post-traumatic adhesions and cruciate damage.

8.6 Degenerative joint disease

Evidence of degenerative change of the joint is commonly present in patients with meniscal lesions as an associated feature. On the other hand, degeneration of the menisci is an almost universal eventual accompaniment of osteoarthrosis of the knee.

Identification of established degenerative joint disease is important in the management of the patient, as its presence may persuade the surgeon to forego the removal of a meniscus, particularly if this is degenerate and not torn.

The presence of osteophytes on the preliminary film is not necessarily sufficient evidence on which to establish the diagnosis of progressive osteoarthrosis. It is not

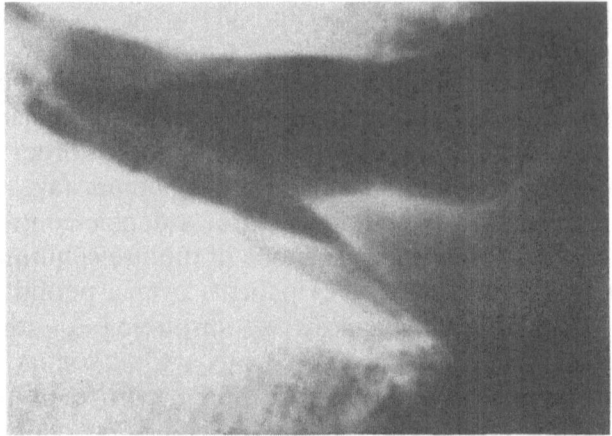

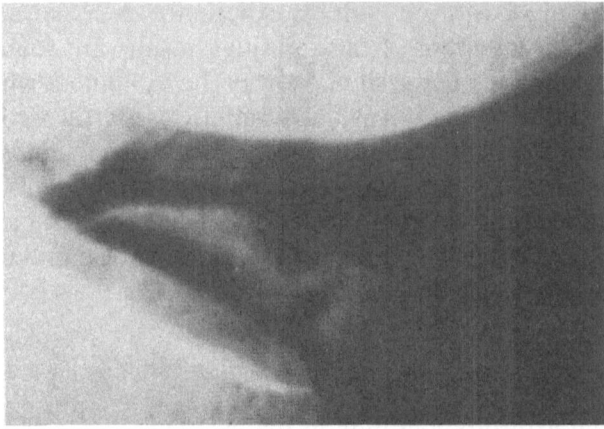

Fig. 8.7 *Tear of posterior horn of medial meniscus.* The patient had had his lateral meniscus removed 17 years earlier at the age of 20. 11 years later an arthrotomy had been performed for the removal of loose bodies. The present symptoms were thought to be related to secondary degenerative joint disease, but arthrography was requested to differentiate between two possible diagnoses – a tear of the medial meniscus and a retained fragment of the lateral meniscus. Arthroscopy showed a large remnant of the lateral posterior horn; the medial meniscus appeared normal in its anterior two-thirds with the suggestion of a split in the posterior horn (which was not, however, clearly visualized). Arthrography also showed the lateral remnant and a vertical tear of the posterior horn of the medial meniscus (lower figure); in the upper illustration, loss of the articular cartilage is shown on the medial femoral condyle.

infrequently that one finds an apparently normal articular cartilage in the presence of marginal osteophytes. Arthrographically, degenerative change is heralded by absorption of positive contrast medium into the surface of the articular cartilage; as the process continues, irregularity of the surface and reduction of the depth of cartilage occurs. Such thinning of articular cartilage is eventually evident on the plain film. Erosion of articular cartilage is often found in relation to a meniscal tear or irregularity (Fig. 8.7). Direct pressure by a torn fragment can clearly damage the articular surface, reinforcing the case for removal of an abnormal meniscus which is sufficiently deformed to cause pressure erosion of the articular cartilage.

Arthrography is rarely employed as a primary diagnostic procedure for degenerative joint disease, but the demonstration of its degree during arthrography sometimes helps the orthopaedic surgeon in the management of a knee derangement in the middle-aged patient. The same is true for the younger patient who, by reason of repeated athletic injury, has a 'middle-aged' knee.

8.7. Ligament injuries

8.7.1. Capsule and medial collateral ligament

Tears of the capsule of the knee joint are common as solitary lesions and in association with meniscal tears. They may be shown arthrographically by the demonstration of leakage of positive-contrast medium into the extracapsular soft tissues (Wang and Marshall, 1975). Such a manifestation depends upon rupture of the synovial lining of the joint. As this may seal effectively in a few days, only acute or recurrent capsular ruptures are usually demonstrated. These may be associated with tears of the integral collateral ligament on the medial side of the joint. Little value is gained from the arthrographic diagnosis of capsular tears; if these are not demonstrable clinically they are probably of trivial degree. An arthrogram does not distinguish a partial from a complete tear of the medial collateral ligament. Only views with forced valgus stress will establish complete rupture and general anaesthesia may be required if the knee is painful; such views are obtained without the need for arthrography.

8.7.2. Cruciate ligaments

The extra-synovial situation of the cruciate ligaments makes their demonstration difficult. As only 12 per cent of Smillie's (1970) 7500 meniscectomy patients had rupture of the anterior cruciate ligament, it might be suggested that one could achieve an 88 per cent diagnostic accuracy if all cruciate ligaments were reported as intact at arthrography. Such a degree of accuracy has not been reported and is certainly outside our experience.

Although frontal intercondylar views have been employed in the study of the cruciate ligaments (Roebuck, 1977), most workers have based their observations on the lateral radiograph of the knee supplementing the technique by positive-contrast methods (Mittler *et al.*, 1972), tomography (Dalinka *et al.*, 1973), 'drawer' manoeuvres (Stoker, 1975) and xerography.

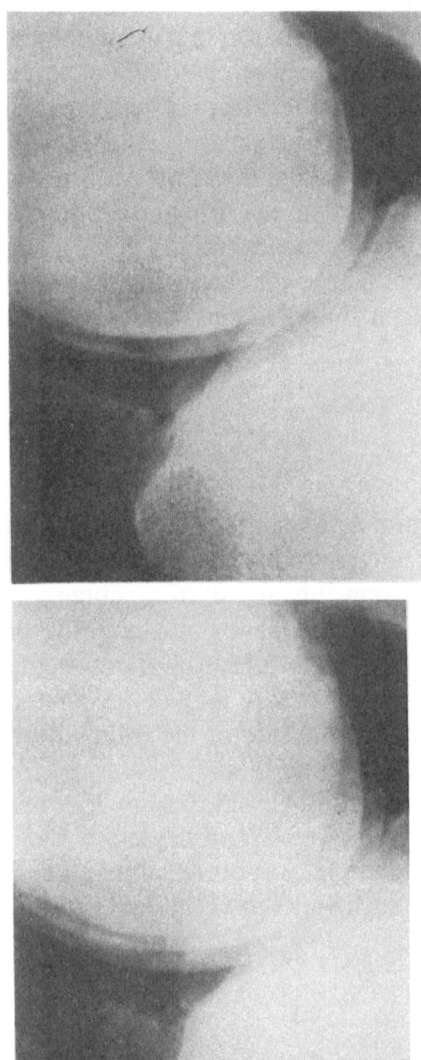

Fig. 8.8 *Ruptured anterior cruciate ligament.* Two views of the knee with and without anterior tibial traction show a similar appearance with no identifiable normal anterior cruciate ligament. The rather lobulated shadow close to the site of tibial attachment of the ligament may represent its remnant. A complete rupture was confirmed at arthrotomy.

Results have not, even in the most optimistic reports (Liljedahl *et al.*, 1965), achieved the accuracy of that obtained in the diagnosis of meniscal lesions. Like other workers, we have been disappointed with the results achieved in cruciate assessment. The diagnosis of rupture depends mainly on the negative observation that the cruciate ligament shadow cannot be demonstrated (Fig. 8.8.) and, less

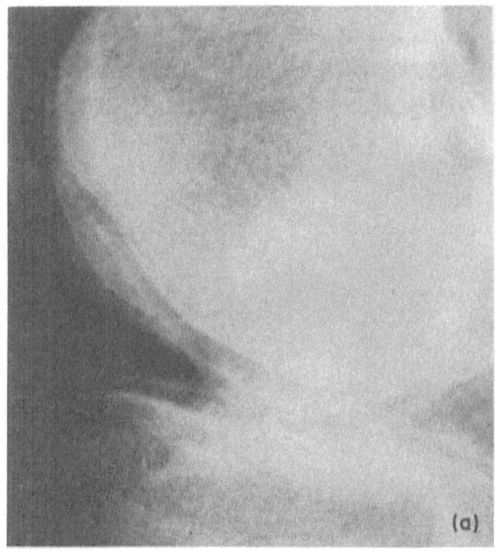

(a)

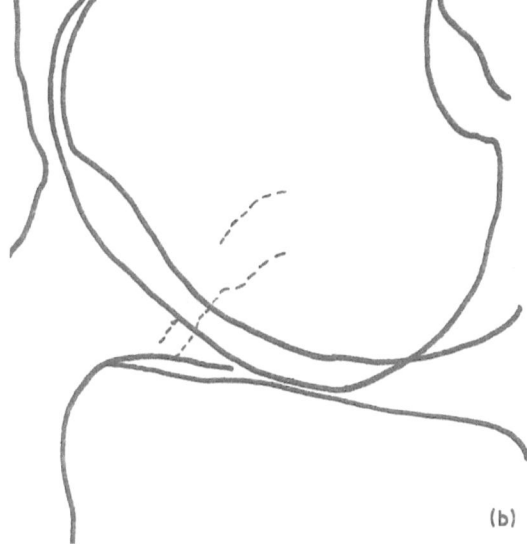

(b)

Fig. 8.9, (a) and (b) *Ruptured anterior cruciate ligament.* In this case, the anterior cruciate ligament shows an ill-defined filling defect which did not straighten under tension (dotted line in (b)). It was found to be ruptured within its intact sheath at operation.

commonly, on the observation of the torn or irregular remnant of the ligament itself (Fig. 8.9). It is perhaps for this reason that arthrographic accuracy is greater in the diagnosis of acute cruciate rupture (Liljedahl *et al.*, 1965). In our practice, not being linked to a sports clinic, we are rarely provided with injured patients early enough to diagnose such lesions. Other centres, with large Accident and Sports Injuries Clinics, are more likely to be successful in this respect.

However, it is unusual for an abnormal anterior cruciate ligament to be entirely normal on the arthrogram. When its anterior border is well shown and straightens with the anterior 'drawer' manoeuvre (Fig. 8.10), it is generally intact. Care must

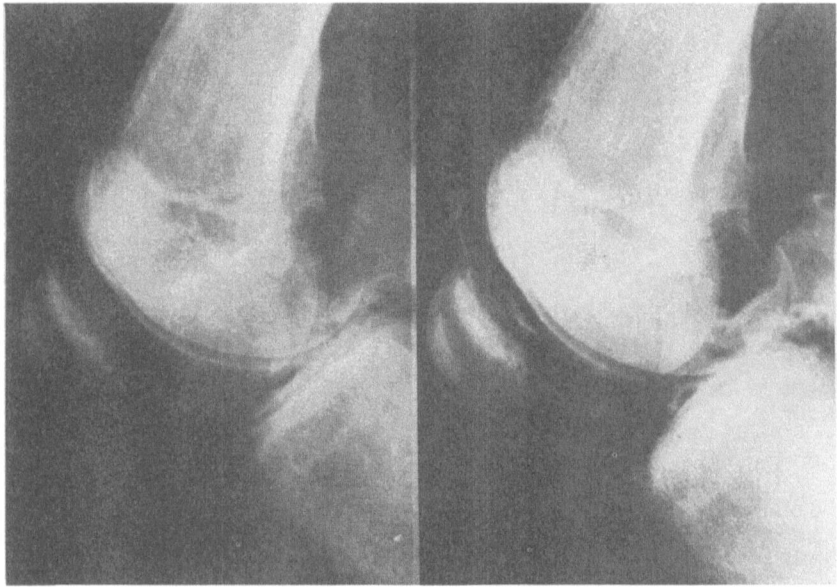

Fig. 8.10 *Normal anterior cruciate demonstrated at arthrography.* Two arthrographic views obtained to demonstrate the normal anterior cruciate ligament. On the left, with the knee relaxed, the anterior margin of the ligament is poorly shown; on the right, a film obtained during the anterior drawer manoeuvre shows that the ligament straightens under tension, confirming its integrity. The margin of the posterior cruciate is also shown, as it produces a tent-like appearance in combination with the anterior cruciate ligament.

be taken to ensure that the observed margin has the anatomical features of the anterior cruciate ligament (Fig. 8.11). Dalinka and Garofola (1976) have emphasized the pitfall of interpreting an anterior synovial fold for the cruciate ligament. Because the ligament is extrasynovial, a false negative diagnosis is certainly possible by the demonstration of an intact synovial fold, containing within it a partially or completely ruptured cruciate ligament.

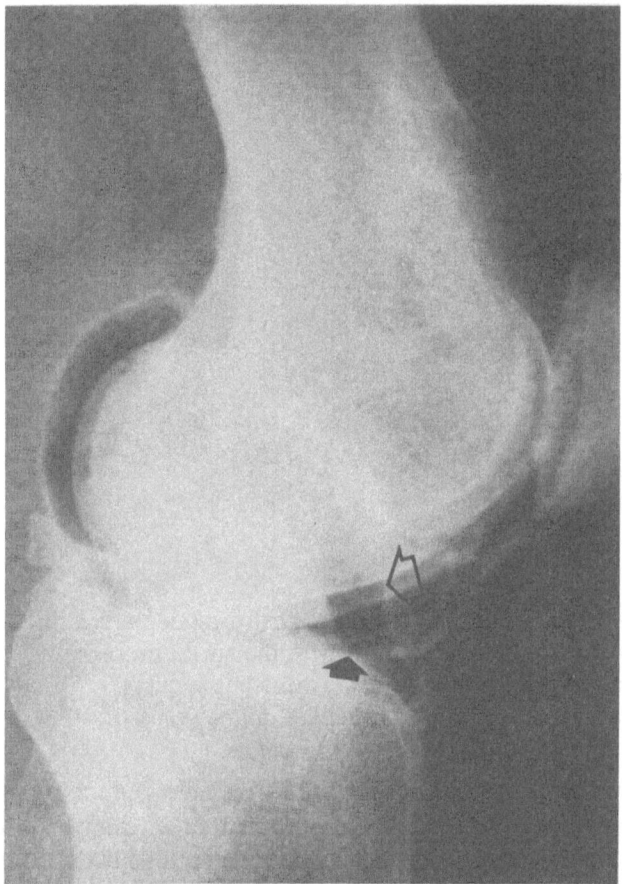

Fig. 8.11 *Normal anterior cruciate ligament.* The
ligament is shown passing into the intercondylar region
from its distal attachment of the tibial plateau (black
arrow). The irregular scalloped-edged filling defect
lying anteriorly (open arrow) is the infrapatellar pad of
fat with its synovial fold.

8.8 Arthrography in other disorders of the knee

8.8.1 Popliteal cysts and other bursal disorders

A popliteal cyst, 'Baker's cyst' (Baker, 1877) is an enlarged gastrocnemio-semimembranosus bursa. Since this bursa is a normal structure, it is impossible to
define exactly what constitutes enlargement. Arthrographically, the bursa either
communicates with the joint and is visualized (Fig. 8.12) or it does not.

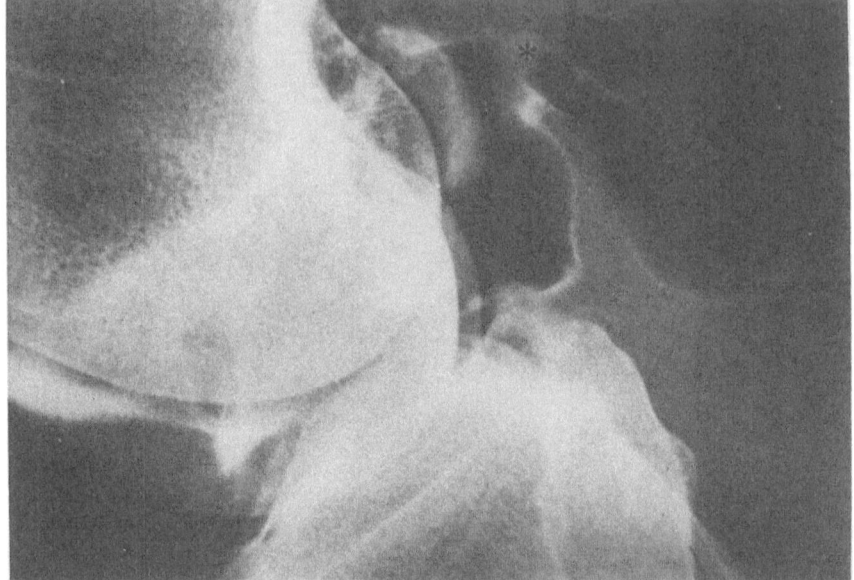

Fig. 8.12 *Gastrocnemio-semimembranosus bursa.* A bursa of small to moderate size has filled during arthrography, the neck of the bursa (*) is evident. Although the presence of such a bursa is not necessarily abnormal, it is often associated with some meniscal abnormality–in this case, a small parrot-beak tear of the lateral meniscus.

Consequently, although some patients complain primarily of a tight palpable cyst behind the knee, others are unaware of its presence. Enlargement of the bursa to any degree depends on the presence at some time of a constant or intermittent joint effusion. Although this of itself could cause enlargement of the bursa *pari passu* with the main joint, such enlargement usually results from its combination with the pumping action of normal flexion and extension of the knee. This forces the joint fluid from the posterior compartment into the bursa, its return being prevented by the valve-like action of the semimembranosus and medial head of the gastrocnemius muscles at the neck of the bursa.

Because of the direct association of the popliteal cyst with joint effusion, it is frequently found in joint disorders such as meniscal injuries and common arthropathies, e.g. rheumatoid arthritis (Good, 1964). Large cysts may dissect and be the cause of calf pain. Alternatively, they may rupture and produce pain, tenderness and swelling, simulating a deep vein thrombosis (Fig. 8.13).

Numerous papers have been written on the differential diagnosis of popliteal cysts before and after rupture, with particular emphasis on the differentiation from deep vein thrombosis. Two major methods of confirming the diagnosis are ultrasonography and arthrography (Meire *et al.*, 1974; Sweet *et al.*, 1975). In such circumstances, arthrography shows the rupture and dissection of the calf tissues by

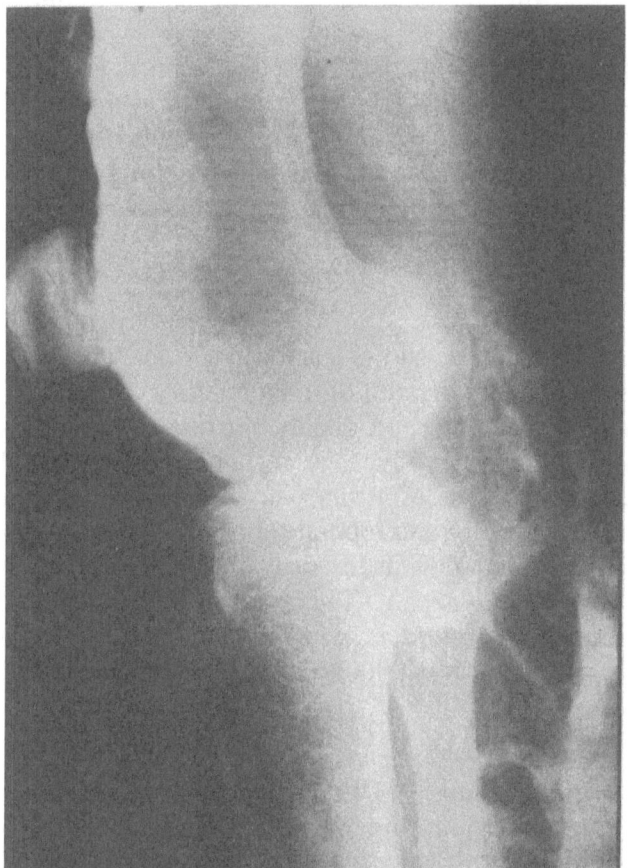

Fig. 8.13 *Ruptured popliteal cyst.* This patient, a
sufferer from chronic rheumatoid arthritis for many
years, presented with a tender swollen calf. Ascending
venography was normal, but the arthrogram shows
passage of the contrast medium into an extensive space
in the calf caused by the rupture of a
gastrocnemio-semimembranosus cyst.

the opacified fluid. Clear anatomical demonstration of such an event has not been
achieved with any regularity in the past by ultrasonography, but it is to be expected
that the better discrimination achieved by modern techniques and equipment will
resolve the problem (Gompels and Darlington, 1979).

Examination by ultrasound has the advantage of being non-invasive, but will not
demonstrate small cysts or necessarily establish that a cyst has ruptured into the
calf. Arthrography, on the other hand, will not demonstrate a cyst which does not
communicate with the joint. A double-contrast technique is to be preferred in these

circumstances as, occasionally, gas will enter the bursa where fluid medium will not.

Certain authors (Meyerding and Van Denmark, 1943; Burleson *et al.*, 1956) believe that many popliteal cysts are the result of posterior herniations through the joint capsule. If the arthrographer has any doubt about whether he is observing a lax posterior capsule or a cyst, fluoroscopy of the knee in the fully extended position will tighten the capsule, but will not obliterate a cyst caused either by a bursa or a herniation.

8.8.2 Inflammatory synovial disorders

On arthrography, normal synovial membrane shows a smooth surface which coats well with water-soluble contrast media. Any irritant or inflammatory condition will alter this appearance, in a non-specific manner, producing blurring of the margins due to absorption of medium into the perisynovial tissue. The thickness of the synovium cannot be measured, as both sides cannot be defined; thickening, however, is indicated by surface irregularity and lobulation at the expense of the synovial cavity. Some of the nodular filling defects in rheumatoid arthritis are due to fibrinous loose bodies ('melon seed bodies') (Taylor and Ansell, 1972). In rheumatoid arthritis, popliteal cysts are found in over 40 per cent of patients (Taylor, 1968) and enlargement of the suprapatellar pouch is a constant finding.

8.8.3 Pigmented villonodular synovitis

In this tumour-like disorder, the gross changes are similar to rheumatoid arthritis, but with greater nodularity of the synovium and numerous recesses and filling defects (Rein *et al.*, 1964). A double-contrast technique delineates the nodular villous protrusions even more strikingly (Wolfe and Guiliano, 1970).

8.8.4 Synovial osteochondromatosis

This rare metaplastic disorder is characterized by the presence of multiple loose bodies, some of which contain calcium or bone. Arthrography will demonstrate radiolucent cartilaginous bodies lying within the expanded synovial cavity, in contradistinction to pigmented villonodular synovitis (Crittenden *et al.*, 1970). The synovial lining in this condition is, however, also nodular to some degree because it is thickened and osteocartilaginous bodies are present in the subsynovial layer. A double-contrast technique is to be preferred for the demonstration of such loose bodies.

8.8.5 Synovial haemangioma

This rare tumour may be diagnosed on the plain film by the combination of synovial swelling and the formation of phleboliths.

An alternative technique of diagnostic importance is thermography, when the lesion is shown to be warm.

As angiomas of joints may lie outside and/or within the synovial cavity, arthrography helps to define the extent of the lesion. Nodular masses of non-specific type are shown (Thomas and Andress, 1972). The combination of arthrography and arteriography establishes the nature of the disorder and its extent (Forrest and Staple, 1971).

8.8.6 Haemophilic arthropathy

Arthrography has been performed in patients suffering from haemophilia (Salerno *et al.*, 1972) and is not contraindicated in patients whose therapy is well-controlled. Such examinations delineate the cartilaginous and bony changes of this disorder. Communicating subchondral cysts are demonstrable, as well as synovial change.

The examination can rarely be justified.

8.8.7 Blount's disease

Arthrography has been reported as a valuable aid in the evaluation and management of Blount's disease (Dalinka *et al.*, 1974), as it permits visualization of the unossified cartilage anlage of the medial plateau. The authors claim that the decision to perform osteotomy and the degree of angular correction can be influenced by such information.

8.8.8 Dysplasia epiphysealis hemimelica

In a similar way, the uncalcified condylar cartilage can be visualized in this rare bone disorder (Goldstein, 1973).

8.8.9 Hypertrophy of the infrapatellar fat pad (Hoffa's pad)

Enlargement of this fat pad may be due to a variety of causes, oedema, hypertrophy or post-traumatic fibrosis. Symptoms secondary to enlargement are caused by entrapment of synovial tags (Smillie, 1970).

Hoffa's disease is, by definition, idiopathic enlargement of this fat pad and is rare. Most enlargements are considered to be secondary to meniscal tears, a discoid meniscus or synovitis (Stenström, 1968). A large infrapatellar fat pad may obscure the anterior horn of the medial meniscus at arthrography.

Enlargement of the fat pad to a degree sufficient to cause locking is extremely rare (Ricklin *et al.*, 1971).

Considerable doubt exists as to whether Hoffa's disease is an entity and the radiologist should demur from making such an arthrographic diagnosis.

8.8.10 Lipoma arborescens

This rare intra-articular tumour has been demonstrated arthrographically (Burgan, 1971). The combination of a soft tissue of fat density of the plain radiograph which proves, on arthrography, to be a nodular intra-articular mass should suggest the diagnosis.

References

Aichroth, P. (1971). Osteochondritis dissecans of the knee. A clinical survey. *Journal of Bone and Joint Surgery*, **53–B**, 440–7.

Anderson, P.W., Harley, J.D. and Maslin P.U. (1976). Arthrographic evaluation of problems with united tibial plateau fractures. *Radiology*, **119**, 75–8.

Anderson, P.W. and Maslin, P. (1974). Tomography applied to knee arthrography. *Radiology*, **110**, 271–5.

Ashby, M.E., Shields, C.L. and Karmy, J.R. (1975). Diagnosis of osteochondral fractures in acute traumatic patellar dislocations using air arthrography. *Journal of Trauma*, **15**, 1032–3.

Baker, W.M. (1877). On the formation of synovial cysts in the leg in connection with disease of the knee joint. *St Bartholomew's Hospital Reports*, **XIII**, 245–61.

Burgan, D.W. (1971). Lipoma arborescens of the knee: another case of filling defects on a knee arthrogram. *Radiology*, **101**, 583–4.

Burleson, R.J., Bickel, W.H. and Dahlin, D.C. (1956). Popliteal cyst: a clinicopathological survey. *Journal of Bone and Joint Surgery*, **38–A**, 1265–74.

Crittenden, J.J., Jones, D.M. and Santarelli, A.G. (1970). Knee arthrogram in synovial chondromatosis. *Radiology*, **94**, 133–4.

Dalinka, M.K., Coren, G.S. and Wershba, M. (1973). Knee arthrography. *C.R.C. Critical Reviews in Clinical Radiology and Nuclear Medicine*, **4**, 1–59.

Dalinka, M.K., Coren, G., Hensinger, R. and Irani, R.N. (1974). Arthrography in Blount's disease. *Radiology*, **113**, 161–4.

Dalinka, M.K. and Garofola, J. (1976). The infrapatellar synovial fold: a cause for confusion in the evaluation of the anterior cruciate ligament. *American Journal of Roentgenology*, **127**, 589–91.

Fordham, S.D. and Turner, A.F. (1976). Arthrography in penetrating injuries. *Journal of the American College of Emergency Physicians*, **5**, 265–7.

Forrest, J. and Staple, T.W (1971). Synovial haemangioma of the knee. Demonstration of arthrography and arteriography. *American Journal of Roentgenology*, **112**, 512–6.

Goldstein, W.B. (1973). Dysplasia epiphysealis hemimelica with confirmation by knee arthrography. *British Journal of Radiology*, **46**, 470–2.

Gompels, B.M. and Darlington, L.G. (1979). Grey scale ultrasonography and arthrography in evaluation of popliteal cysts. *Clinical Radiology*, **30**, 539–45.

Good, A.E. (1964). Rheumatoid arthritis, Baker's cyst and 'thrombophlebitis'. *Arthritis and Rheumatism*, **7**, 56–64.

Horns, J.W. (1977). The diagnosis of chondromalacia by double contrast arthrography of the knee. *Journal of Bone and Joint Surgery*, **59–A**, 119–20.

Liljedahl, S.-O., Lindvall, N. and Wetterfors, J. (1965). Early diagnosis and treatment of acute ruptures of the anterior cruciate ligament. *Journal of Bone and Joint Surgery,* **47-A**, 1503–13.

Lindblom, K. (1938). The arthrographic appearance of the ligaments of the knee joint. *Acta Radiologica,* **19**, 582–600.

Meire, H., Lindsay, D.J., Swinson, D.R. and Hamilton, E.B. (1974). Comparison of ultrasound and positive contrast arthrography in the diagnosis of popliteal and calf swellings. *Annals of the Rheumatic Diseases,* **33**, 408, 221–4.

Meyerding, H.W. and Van Denmark, R.E. (1943). Posterior hernia of the knee (Baker's cyst, popliteal cyst, semimembranosus bursitis, medial gastrocnemius bursitis and popliteal bursitis). *Journal of the American Medical Association,* **122**, 858.

Mittler, S., Freiberger, R.H. and Harrison-Stubbs, M. (1972). A method of improving cruciate ligament visualization in double-contrast arthrography. *Radiology,* **102**, 441–2.

Nicholas, J.A., Freiberger, R.H. and Killoran, P.J. (1970). Double-contrast arthrography of the knee. Its value in the management of 225 knee derangements. *Journal of Bone and Joint Surgery,* **52-A**, 203–20.

Rein, B.I., Bilodeau, L.P. and Johanson, P. (1964). Arthrography and arteriography in pigmented villonodular synovitis of the knee. *American Journal of Roentgenology,* **92**, 1322–7.

Ricklin, P., Rüttimann, A. and Del Buono, M.S. (1971). *Meniscus Lesions,* Thieme Verlag, Stuttgart.

Roebuck, E.J. (1977). Double contrast knee arthrography. Some new points of technique including the use of Dimer X. *Clinical Radiology,* **28**, 247–57.

Salerno, N.R., Menges, J.F. and Borns, P.F. (1972). Arthrograms in hemophilia. *Radiology,* **102**, 135–8.

Smillie, I.S. (1970). *Injuries of the knee joint,* 4th Edn. Livingstone, Edinburgh.

Staple, T.W. (1972). Extra-meniscal lesions demonstrated by double-contrast arthrography of the knee. *Radiology,* **102**, 311–9.

Stenström, R. (1968). Arthrography of the knee joint in children. Roentgenologic anatomy, diagnosis and the use of multiple discriminant analysis. *Acta Radiologica Supplement,* **281**, 47.

Stoker, D.J. (1975). Double contrast arthrography of the knee in the diagnosis of meniscus injury. *X-ray Focus,* **14**, 26–34.

Swett, H.A., Jaffe, R.B. and McIff, E.B. (1975). Popliteal cysts: presentation as thombophlebitis. *Radiology,* **115**, 613–5.

Taylor, A.R. (1969). Arthrography of the knee in rheumatoid arthritis. *British Journal of Radiology,* **42**, 493–7.

Taylor, A.R., and Ansell, B.M. (1972). Arthrography of the knee before and after synovectomy for rheumatoid arthritis. *Journal of Bone and Joint Surgery,* **54-B**, 110–5.

Thijn, C.J.P. (1979). *Arthrography of the knee joint,* p. 61–5. Springer-Verlag, Berlin, Heidelberg, New York.

Thomas, M.L. and Andress, M.R. (1972). Angioma of the knee demonstrated by angiography and arthrography. Report of a case. *Acta Radiologica,* **12**, 217–20.

Wang, J.B. and Marshall, J.L. (1975). Acute ligamentous injuries of the knee. Single contrast arthrography–a diagnostic aid. *Journal of Trauma,* **15**, 431–40.

Wershba, M., Dalinka, M.K., Coren, G.S. and Cotler, J. (1975). Double contrast knee arthrography in the evaluation of osteochondritis dissecans. *Clinical Orthopedics*, **107**, 81–6.

Wolfe, R.D. and Guiliano, V.J. (1970). Double-contrast arthrography in the diagnosis of pigmented villonodular synovitis of the knee. *American Journal of Roentgenology*, **110**, 793–9.

Index